Dr. Fahad is an exceptionally intelligent and diligent physician, holding dual majors and embodying a helpful, fast-learning person. He stands out for his remarkable intellect and tireless work ethic in the medical field. Juggling dual specializations, he efficiently lends his assistance while rapidly absorbing knowledge.

As an educator, Dr. Fahad demonstrates a remarkable ability to impart knowledge and offer substantial aid. He's an incredibly impressive teacher, enriching minds and profoundly impacting his students. His exceptional capacity to convey information directly and effectively makes him an outstanding educator.

Dr. Fahad epitomizes diligence and a passion for learning, serving as a symbol of effective teaching and excellence in medicine. These qualities render him a revered and respected figure in the medical community, eliciting admiration and esteem from all quarters.

Dr. Fahad Mudhhi AlOtaibi

SURGERY MADE SIMPLE

Quick review for more than 200 Diseases in General Surgery

AUSTIN MACAULEY PUBLISHERS
LONDON * CAMBRIDGE * NEW YORK * SHARJAH

Copyright © Dr. Fahad Mudhhi AlOtaibi 2024

The right of Dr. Fahad Mudhhi AlOtaibi to be identified as author of this work has been asserted by the author in accordance with Federal Law No. (7) of UAE, Year 2002, Concerning Copyrights and Neighboring Rights.

All rights reserved. No part of this publication may be reproduced, stored in a retrieval system, or transmitted in any form or by any means, electronic, mechanical, photocopying, recording, or otherwise, without the prior permission of the publishers.

Any person who commits any unauthorized act in relation to this publication may be liable to legal prosecution and civil claims for damages.

ISBN – 9789948747239 – (Paperback)
ISBN – 9789948747246 – (E-Book)

Application Number: MC-10-01-5345781
Age Classification: E

The age group that matches the content of the books has been classified according to the age classification system issued by the UAE Media Council.

Printer Name: iPrint Global Ltd
Printer Address: Witchford, England

First Published 2024
AUSTIN MACAULEY PUBLISHERS FZE
Sharjah Publishing City
P.O Box [519201]
Sharjah, UAE
www.austinmacauley.ae
+971 655 95 202

Table of Contents

Introduction	17
Terminology	19
Abdominal Aortic Aneurysm (AAA)	32
Abdominal Compartment Syndrome	33
Abdominal or Retroperitoneal Sarcoma	34
Abdominal Trauma	35
Abdominal Wall Hernia	36
Accessory Spleen Removal	37
Achalasia	38
Acute Cholecystitis	39
Acute Perforated Peptic Ulcer	40
Adenoid Cystic Carcinoma	41
Adrenal Adenoma	42
Adrenal Hemorrhage	43
Adrenal Incidentaloma	44
Adrenal Insufficiency (Addison's Disease)	45
Adrenal Myelolipoma	46
Ameloblastoma	47
Ampullary Cancer	48

Anal Abscess and Fistula	49
Anal Cancer	50
Anal Fissures	51
Aortic Aneurysm	52
Aortoenteric Fistula	53
Aortoiliac Occlusive Disease	54
Appendiceal Abscess	55
Appendiceal Carcinoid Tumor	56
Appendiceal Goblet Cell Carcinoma	57
Appendiceal Mucocele	58
Appendicitis	59
Arterial Embolism	60
Arteriovenous Fistula	61
Bariatric Surgery	62
Benign Prostatic Hyperplasia (BPH)	72
Biliary Colic	73
Biliary Tract Disorders	74
Bleeding Esophageal Varices	75
Boerhaave Syndrome	76
Bowel Perforation	77
Breast Cancer	78
Bronchiectasis	79
Bronchopulmonary Dysplasia (BPD)	80
Bronchopulmonary Sequestration	81

Carotid Artery Disease	82
Cecal Volvulus	83
Celiac Artery Compression Syndrome (Median Arcuate Ligament Syndrome)	84
Chest Wall Tumors	85
Cholangiocarcinoma	87
Cholecystitis	88
Choledochal Cyst	89
Choledocholithiasis	90
Chronic Mesenteric Ischemia	91
Chronic Pancreatitis	92
Chylothorax	93
Chylous Ascites	94
Colon Cancer	95
Colorectal Cancer	96
Colorectal Polyps	97
Cystic Adventitial Disease	98
Deep Vein Thrombosis (DVT)	99
Desmoid Tumor	100
Diaphragmatic Hernia	101
Diverticulitis	102
Diverticulosis	103
Ectopic Pregnancy	104
Empyema	105

Esophageal Cancer	106
Esophageal Stricture	107
Esophageal Varices	108
Fecal Incontinence	109
Femoral Hernia	110
Foreign Body Ingestion	111
Fournier's Gangrene	112
Gallbladder Cancer	113
Gallbladder Polyps	114
Gallstone Ileus	115
Gallstone Pancreatitis	116
Gallstones (Cholelithiasis) and Cholecystitis	117
Gastric Cancer	118
Gastric Leiomyosarcoma	119
Gastric Ulcer	120
Gastroesophageal Reflux Disease (GERD)	121
Gastrointestinal Bleeding	122
Gastrointestinal Fistula	123
Gastrointestinal or Abdominal Lymphoma	124
Gastrointestinal Stromal Tumor (GIST)	125
Gastroparesis	126
Giant Cell Tumor of Bone	127
Hemorrhoids	128
Hepatic Abscess	129

Hepatic Hemangioma	130
Hepatic Hydatid Cyst	131
Hernias	132
Hiatal Hernia	133
Hidradenitis Suppurativa	134
Hirschsprung's Disease	135
Hydrocele	136
Hydronephrosis	137
Hyperparathyroidism-Jaw Tumor Syndrome	138
Incarcerated Hernia	139
Inflammatory Bowel Disease (IBD)	140
Inguinal Hernia	141
Intestinal Ischemia	142
Intestinal Lymphangiectasia	143
Intestinal Obstruction in Neonates	144
Intrabdominal Abscess	145
Irritable Bowel Syndrome (IBS)	146
Ischemic Colitis	147
Islet Cell Tumor (Pancreatic Neuroendocrine Tumor)	148
Kawasaki Disease	149
Klippel-Trenaunay Syndrome	150
Langerhans Cell Histiocytosis	151
Leriche Syndrome	152
Lipomas	153

Liver Abscess	**154**
Lung Abscess	**155**
Lung Cancer	**156**
Lymphedema	**157**
Lymphoepithelial Cyst	**158**
Malignant Melanoma	**159**
Mastitis	**160**
May-Thurner Syndrome	**161**
Meckel's Diverticulum	**162**
Mediastinal Tumors	**163**
Mediastinitis	**164**
Mesenteric Ischemia	**165**
Mesothelioma	**166**
Mycotic Aneurysm	**167**
Nasopharyngeal Carcinoma	**168**
Necrotizing Enterocolitis (NEC)	**169**
Necrotizing Fasciitis	**170**
Necrotizing Soft Tissue Infections	**171**
Neuroblastoma	**172**
Neuroendocrine Tumors	**173**
Ovarian Cyst	**174**
Paget-Schroetter Syndrome (Effort Thrombosis)	**175**
Pancreatic Cancer	**176**
Pancreatic Pseudocyst	**177**

Pancreatitis	**178**
Parathyroid Adenoma	**179**
Parathyroid Cancer	**180**
Parathyroid Disorders	**181**
Parathyroid Hyperplasia	**182**
Partial Splenectomy	**183**
Pectus Excavatum	**185**
Pelvic Organ Prolapse	**186**
Peptic Ulcers	**187**
Perianal Abscess	**188**
Peripheral Artery Disease (PAD)	**189**
Peritonitis	**190**
Pilonidal Cyst	**191**
Pilonidal Disease	**192**
Pleural Effusion	**193**
Pleuroparenchymal Fibroelastosis (PPFE)	**194**
Pneumothorax	**195**
Polycystic Liver Disease	**196**
Popliteal Artery Aneurysm	**197**
Popliteal Artery Entrapment Syndrome	**198**
Portal Hypertension	**199**
Primary Spontaneous Pneumothorax	**200**
Pseudomyxoma Peritonei	**201**
Pulmonary Embolism	**202**

Pulmonary Fibrosis	203
Pulmonary Sequestration	204
Pyloric Stenosis	205
Raynaud's Disease	206
Rectal Cancer	207
Rectal Prolapse	208
Renal Artery Stenosis	209
Renal Stones (Nephrolithiasis)	210
Retroperitoneal Fibrosis	211
Ruptured Abdominal Aortic Aneurysm (AAA)	212
Small Bowel Obstruction	213
Spigelian Hernia	214
Spleen Biopsy	215
Splenectomy	216
Splenic Disorders	218
Splenic Rupture	219
Splenopexy	220
Splenorenal Shunt	221
Splenorrhaphy	223
Splenosis Resection	224
Splenunculi Removal	225
Strangulated Hernia	226
Superior Mesenteric Artery Syndrome (SMAS)	227
Surgical Emphysema	228

Surgical Site Infection (SSI)	229
Thoracic Aortic Aneurysm	230
Thoracic Endovascular Aortic Repair (TEVAR)	231
Thoracic Outlet Syndrome (TOS)	232
Thromboangiitis Obliterans (Buerger's Disease)	233
Thrombosed Hemorrhoids	234
Thymic Hyperplasia	235
Thymoma	236
Thyroid Cancer	237
Thyroid Disorders	238
Thyroid Nodules	239
Tracheal Stenosis	240
Tracheoesophageal Fistula	241
Tuberculosis (Pulmonary Tuberculosis)	242
Varicose Veins	243
Vascular Trauma	244
Ventral Hernia	245
Volvulus	246
Wilms Tumor (Nephroblastoma)	247
Zenker's Diverticulum	248

Author's statement

Surgery Made Simple: Quick Review for more than 200 Diseases in General Surgery

In the intricate world of surgery, where every incision holds the promise of healing, knowledge is the linchpin upon which medical mastery rests. It is this understanding that has inspired the creation of " Surgery Made Simple: Quick Review for more than 200 Diseases in General Surgery" This handbook is not just a compendium of medical wisdom; it is a guiding light for the medical students venturing into the complexities of surgical sciences.

Embarking on a Journey Through Surgical Knowledge

Within the pages of "Surgery Made Simple," a fascinating odyssey awaits. Imagine a handbook that doesn't just inundate you with complex medical terminology but gently guides you through the labyrinth of more than 200 common surgical diseases. It is designed to be your trusted companion, offering clear and concise insights into the intricacies of ailments that surgeons encounter in their daily practice.

Demystifying Complexity, One Page at a Time

What sets "Surgery Made Simple" apart is its commitment to simplicity. Each page is a treasure trove of essential information, distilling the complexities of diseases into digestible facts. Whether you are a novice medical student or a seasoned practitioner seeking quick references, this handbook is tailored to meet your needs. It is a bridge between theoretical knowledge and practical application, ensuring that the path to surgical expertise is not marred by confusion.

A Gateway to Deeper Understanding

While "Surgery Made Simple" offers a comprehensive overview of more than 200 diseases, it is important to note that this handbook serves as a gateway. The complexities of the human body and the nuances of surgical interventions are vast. For those seeking a deeper understanding or exploring specialized areas, the references within the book provide a roadmap. Delve into the world of surgical literature, learn from pioneers in the field, and expand your knowledge beyond the confines of this handbook.

In essence, " Surgery Made Simple: Quick Review for more than 200 Diseases in General Surgery" is not just a book; it is a key that unlocks the doors to surgical wisdom. It is an invitation to explore, learn, and ultimately, contribute meaningfully to the art and science of surgery. So, open its pages, absorb its knowledge, and let it be your compass as you navigate the intricate world of surgical medicine. Your journey to mastering surgery starts here.

Introduction

The Symphony of Surgery: Celebrating the Unsung Heroes of the Surgical Team

In the hushed and sterile environment of the operating room, where every moment counts, a symphony of skill, precision, and dedication unfolds. At the heart of this orchestrated performance stands the surgical team, a group of unsung heroes whose seamless collaboration turns the daunting challenge of surgery into a harmonious art form.

The Surgical Maestro: The Surgeon

The surgeon, akin to the conductor of an orchestra, leads the team with expertise honed through years of training and experience. Their hands are steady, their decisions swift, navigating the delicate balance between cutting-edge techniques and time-tested methods. With a profound understanding of the human body, they guide the team through the intricate dance of surgery, ensuring each movement serves the ultimate purpose: the well-being of the patient.

The Healing Hands: Surgical Assistants and Nurses

Beside the surgeon are the skilled hands of surgical assistants and nurses, the virtuosos who anticipate every need, ensuring a seamless procedure. Their role is multi-faceted, from passing instruments with precision to providing comforting words to the patient. They are the pillars upon which the surgeon leans, their expertise enhancing the entire surgical process.

The Guardians of Safety: Anesthetists and Technicians

Invisible yet essential, anesthetists maintain the delicate balance between keeping the patient pain-free and ensuring they wake up safely after the surgery.

Their vigilant watch over vital signs is the bedrock of a successful procedure. Meanwhile, technicians manage the intricate technology, from advanced imaging systems to robotic surgical tools, ensuring that the surgeon's vision is brought to life with unmatched accuracy.

The Compassionate Communicators: Surgical Counsellors

Beyond the operating table, surgical counselors provide a vital link between the medical team and the patient's family. They translate complex medical jargon into understandable information, offering solace and reassurance during moments of anxiety. Their compassion and empathy create a bridge of understanding, fostering trust and confidence among concerned loved ones.

The Unsung Symphony

Together, these individuals form the unsung symphony of the surgical world. Their collective expertise, dedication, and tireless commitment to the welfare of their patients create a legacy of healing. Every successful surgery is a testament to their collaboration, a testament to the countless hours of training, and a testament to their unwavering passion for medicine.

In the world of surgery, where every procedure is a high-stakes performance, the surgical team stands as a beacon of hope and healing. Their collective efforts not only transform lives but also exemplify the extraordinary power of teamwork, reminding us that in the hands of these skilled professionals, the art of surgery truly becomes a masterpiece of humanity.

Terminology

1. **Anesthesia:** Loss of sensation, with or without loss of consciousness, especially as induced by an anesthetic substance.
2. **Incision:** A cut made in body tissues during surgery, often to access a part of the body.
3. **Suture:** Stitching of a wound or incision by sewing the edges together with thread or wire.
4. **Hemorrhage:** Excessive bleeding, often a concern during surgery.
5. **Ligation:** The process of tying off blood vessels or ducts to prevent bleeding or the flow of fluids.
6. **Graft:** Tissue or an organ transplanted from a donor site to a recipient site.
7. **Laparoscopy:** A minimally invasive surgical technique involving small incisions and a camera to view and treat abdominal or pelvic organs.
8. **Biopsy:** Removal of a small piece of tissue for examination, usually to diagnose diseases like cancer.
9. **Cauterization:** The use of heat or chemicals to treat a wound or injury, often to stop bleeding or remove abnormal tissue.
10. **Sepsis:** A potentially life-threatening condition caused by the body's response to an infection, which can occur after surgery if bacteria enter the bloodstream.
11. **Laparotomy**: A large surgical incision into the abdominal cavity, often to explore or perform procedures on abdominal organs.
12. **Hemostasis**: The process of stopping bleeding, often achieved through various surgical techniques.
13. **Cautery**: The use of heat or electricity to remove or close off a part of the body, such as a blood vessel, to prevent bleeding.

14. **Debridement**: The removal of damaged or dead tissue from a wound to promote healing.
15. **Laser surgery**: Surgery that uses a laser beam to cut, remove, or destroy tissue.
16. **Suturing**: The act of stitching a wound or incision to promote healing and prevent infection.
17. **Fasciotomy**: Surgical cutting of the fascia, the connective tissue surrounding muscles, to relieve tension or pressure.
18. **Embolectomy**: Surgical removal of an embolus, a blood clot, or foreign material blocking a blood vessel.
19. **Resection**: The removal of all or part of an organ, tissue, or structure during surgery.
20. **Sterilization**: The process of making an object or area free of all living microorganisms, often crucial in surgical procedures to prevent infections.
21. **Endoscopy**: A medical procedure that uses a thin, flexible tube with a light and camera to visualize the interior of organs or cavities.
22. **Aspiration**: The withdrawal of fluid from a cyst or a tumor, or the suctioning of fluids from the body, such as during a bronchoscopy.
23. **Anastomosis**: The surgical connection between two structures, such as blood vessels or bowel segments.
24. **Catheterization**: The insertion of a thin tube (catheter) into a body cavity or blood vessel to drain fluids, administer treatment, or measure various parameters.
25. **Excision**: The surgical removal of a tumor, tissue, or organ.
26. **Osteotomy**: The surgical cutting of a bone, often performed to correct deformities or to change the bone's alignment.
27. **Gastrostomy**: The creation of an opening into the stomach, usually for inserting a feeding tube.
28. **Laminectomy**: Surgical removal of the bony arch of a vertebra, often to relieve pressure on the spinal cord or nerves.
29. **Tracheostomy**: Surgical creation of an opening in the windpipe (trachea) to assist breathing, commonly done in emergencies or for patients requiring long-term ventilator support.

30. **Arthroscopy**: A minimally invasive surgical procedure in which a small camera is inserted into a joint, allowing visualization and treatment of various joint conditions.
31. **Cholecystectomy**: Surgical removal of the gallbladder, often performed due to gallstones or gallbladder disease.
32. **Colostomy**: Surgical creation of an opening in the colon through the abdominal wall, allowing the passage of stool into a bag outside the body.
33. **Laparoscopic Cholecystectomy**: Minimally invasive surgery to remove the gallbladder using small incisions and a camera.
34. **Thoracotomy**: Surgical incision into the chest wall to access the lungs, heart, or other thoracic structures.
35. **Craniotomy**: Surgical opening of the skull to access the brain, often performed for tumor removal or to treat neurological conditions.
36. **Splenectomy**: Surgical removal of the spleen, typically done to treat certain blood disorders or after traumatic injury.
37. **Cesarean Section (C-section)**: Surgical delivery of a baby through an incision in the mother's abdomen and uterus, performed when a vaginal delivery is not possible or safe.
38. **Hysterectomy**: Surgical removal of the uterus, a procedure commonly performed to treat conditions like uterine cancer or severe uterine bleeding.
39. **Amputation**: Surgical removal of a limb or part of a limb, often necessary due to injury, infection, or disease.
40. **Angioplasty**: Minimally invasive procedure to widen narrowed or obstructed arteries, usually involving the insertion of a balloon catheter to expand the vessel and improve blood flow.
41. **Fasciectomy**: Surgical removal of the fascia, a connective tissue covering muscles, often done to treat conditions like Dupuytren's contracture.
42. **Nephrectomy**: Surgical removal of a kidney, performed due to conditions such as kidney cancer or severe kidney damage.
43. **Circumcision**: Surgical removal of the foreskin covering the head of the penis, often done for cultural, religious, or medical reasons.
44. **Oophorectomy**: Surgical removal of one or both ovaries, usually performed to treat ovarian cancer or other ovarian diseases.

45. **Tonsillectomy**: Surgical removal of the tonsils, often done to treat recurrent tonsillitis or breathing problems.
46. **Coronary Artery Bypass Graft (CABG) Surgery**: A surgical procedure to improve blood flow to the heart by bypassing blocked arteries, typically using blood vessels from other parts of the body.
47. **Cystectomy**: Surgical removal of the bladder, usually performed to treat bladder cancer.
48. **Prostatectomy**: Surgical removal of the prostate gland, commonly done to treat prostate cancer.
49. **Thyroidectomy**: Surgical removal of the thyroid gland, performed to treat thyroid cancer, hyperthyroidism, or large thyroid nodules.
50. **Aneurysm Repair**: A surgical procedure to repair a weakened or bulging blood vessel (aneurysm) to prevent rupture, commonly performed in the aorta or brain arteries.
51. **Mastectomy**: Surgical removal of the breast tissue, often performed as a treatment for breast cancer.
52. **Gastrectomy**: Surgical removal of all or part of the stomach, typically done to treat stomach cancer or severe ulcers.
53. **Laminoplasty**: A surgical procedure to create more space within the spinal canal by cutting the lamina of the vertebra, often done to treat spinal stenosis.
54. **Myringotomy**: Surgical incision into the eardrum to relieve pressure or drain fluid from the middle ear, commonly done to treat chronic ear infections.
55. **Neuroplasty**: Surgical repair or reconstruction of a nerve, often performed to relieve pressure on a compressed nerve or treat nerve injuries.
56. **Pancreatectomy**: Surgical removal of all or part of the pancreas, usually performed to treat pancreatic cancer or severe pancreatitis.
57. **Carpal Tunnel Release**: A surgical procedure to relieve pressure on the median nerve in the wrist, commonly done to treat carpal tunnel syndrome.
58. **Vasectomy**: Surgical procedure for male sterilization, involving the cutting or blocking of the vas deferens to prevent the passage of sperm.

59. **Circumferential Abdominoplasty**: A surgical procedure also known as a body lift, involving the removal of excess skin and fat from the abdomen, hips, and back, often performed after significant weight loss.
60. **Nissen Fundoplication**: Surgical procedure to treat gastroesophageal reflux disease (GERD) by wrapping the top of the stomach around the lower esophagus to prevent stomach acid from flowing back into the esophagus.
61. **Trabeculectomy**: A surgical procedure to create a new drainage channel in the eye for the treatment of glaucoma, a condition characterized by increased intraocular pressure.
62. **Whipple Procedure**: Surgical removal of the head of the pancreas, the duodenum, a portion of the common bile duct, and sometimes the gallbladder, often performed to treat pancreatic cancer.
63. **Ventriculoperitoneal Shunt**: Surgical procedure to treat hydrocephalus, a condition in which there is an abnormal accumulation of cerebrospinal fluid in the brain, by draining excess fluid from the brain into the abdominal cavity.
64. **Hip Replacement (Total Hip Arthroplasty)**: A surgical procedure to replace a damaged or diseased hip joint with an artificial joint made of metal, ceramic, or plastic components.
65. **Corneal Transplant**: A surgical procedure to replace a damaged or diseased cornea with healthy donor tissue, often performed to improve vision in conditions like keratoconus or corneal scarring.
66. **Lobectomy**: Surgical removal of one of the lobes of an organ, most commonly used to refer to the removal of a lobe of the lung or thyroid gland.
67. **Ileostomy**: A surgical procedure to create an opening in the abdominal wall through which a portion of the ileum (part of the small intestine) is brought outside the body, allowing waste to exit the body into an ostomy bag.
68. **Peripheral Vascular Bypass**: A surgical procedure to reroute blood flow around a blocked artery in the peripheral vascular system, typically using a graft to restore proper blood circulation.
69. **Ureteroscopy**: Minimally invasive procedure using a thin tube to remove or break up kidney stones lodged in the ureter or kidney.

70. **Arthroplasty**: Surgical reconstruction or replacement of a joint, commonly done in joints like the knee, hip, or shoulder to relieve pain and improve function, especially in cases of arthritis.
71. **Cervical Cerclage**: A surgical procedure in which a stitch is placed around the cervix during pregnancy to prevent premature birth or miscarriage.
72. **Cystoscopy**: A medical procedure using a thin tube with a camera to examine the interior of the bladder and urinary tract, often used to diagnose urinary problems.
73. **Laminectomy**: Surgical removal of the lamina, a part of the vertebral bone, to relieve pressure on the spinal cord or nerves, commonly performed for spinal stenosis.
74. **MVR (Mitral Valve Replacement)**: A surgical procedure to replace a damaged or diseased mitral valve in the heart with a mechanical or biological valve.
75. **Nissen Fundoplication**: Surgical procedure to treat gastroesophageal reflux disease (GERD) by wrapping the top of the stomach around the lower esophagus to prevent acid reflux.
76. **Orchiectomy**: Surgical removal of one or both testicles, often performed as a treatment for testicular cancer.
77. **Pancreas Transplant**: A surgical procedure to replace a diseased pancreas with a healthy pancreas from a deceased donor, often performed for patients with diabetes.
78. **Septoplasty**: A surgical procedure to straighten the nasal septum, commonly done to improve breathing in individuals with a deviated septum.
79. **Vasovasostomy**: A surgical procedure to reverse a vasectomy, reconnecting the vas deferens to restore the flow of sperm.
80. **Splenorrhaphy**: Surgical repair of a damaged spleen, preserving the organ whenever possible after injury.
81. **Mastoidectomy**: Surgical removal of the mastoid bone in the skull, often performed to treat chronic ear infections or mastoiditis.
82. **Myomectomy**: Surgical removal of uterine fibroids (non-cancerous growths in the uterus) while preserving the uterus, commonly performed for women with fertility issues or heavy menstrual bleeding.

83. **Parathyroidectomy**: Surgical removal of one or more parathyroid glands, usually to treat hyperparathyroidism, a condition where these glands produce excessive parathyroid hormone.
84. **Proctocolectomy**: Surgical removal of the rectum and colon, often performed in cases of inflammatory bowel disease (such as ulcerative colitis) or familial adenomatous polyposis.
85. **Synovectomy**: Surgical removal of the synovial membrane, which lines the joints, often done to treat conditions like rheumatoid arthritis or synovial sarcoma.
86. **Thrombectomy**: Surgical removal of a blood clot from a blood vessel, commonly performed in cases of deep vein thrombosis (DVT) or stroke.
87. **Pancreaticoduodenectomy (Whipple Procedure)**: Surgical removal of the head of the pancreas, the duodenum, and other surrounding structures, often used to treat pancreatic cancer.
88. **Sclerotherapy**: A medical procedure in which a chemical solution is injected into blood vessels or lymphatic vessels to treat conditions like varicose veins or lymphedema.
89. **Stereotactic Surgery**: A minimally invasive surgical technique that uses three-dimensional coordinates to precisely locate and treat abnormalities within the body, often used in brain and breast surgeries.
90. **Thoracentesis**: A medical procedure in which a needle or catheter is inserted into the pleural space (between the lungs and the chest wall) to remove excess fluid or air, commonly used to diagnose or treat pleural effusion.
91. **Otoplasty**: A surgical procedure to reshape the ears, often performed to correct prominent or misshapen ears.
92. **Phlebectomy**: Surgical removal of varicose veins through small incisions, usually done in outpatient settings.
93. **Cholecystostomy**: Surgical creation of an opening in the gallbladder, often done to drain bile in cases of acute cholecystitis.
94. **Panniculectomy**: Surgical removal of excess skin and fat from the lower abdomen, often performed after significant weight loss.
95. **Hemithyroidectomy**: Surgical removal of half of the thyroid gland, typically performed to treat thyroid nodules or thyroid cancer.

96. **Sacroiliac Joint Fusion**: A surgical procedure to stabilize the sacroiliac joint, commonly done to treat chronic lower back pain.
97. **Hypospadias Repair**: Surgical correction of a congenital condition where the opening of the urethra is on the underside of the penis instead of the tip.
98. **Esophagectomy**: Surgical removal of a portion of or the entire esophagus, often done to treat esophageal cancer.
99. **Esophagogastroduodenoscopy (EGD)**: Diagnostic procedure using a flexible tube with a camera to examine the esophagus, stomach, and upper part of the small intestine.
100. **Ventral Hernia Repair**: A surgical procedure to repair a hernia in the abdominal wall, often involving the use of mesh to reinforce the weakened area.
101. **Distal Pancreatectomy**: Surgical removal of the tail or part of the pancreas, often performed to treat pancreatic tumors or chronic pancreatitis.
102. **Chordotomy**: A surgical procedure involving the cutting of specific spinal nerve fibers to relieve severe pain, often used in cancer patients with intractable pain.
103. **Splenorenal Shunt**: Surgical connection between the spleen and the renal vein, used to treat complications of portal hypertension, such as bleeding varices.
104. **Salpingectomy**: Surgical removal of one or both fallopian tubes, often performed for sterilization or to treat conditions like ectopic pregnancy.
105. **Tendon Repair**: A surgical procedure to reattach or repair a torn or damaged tendon, commonly performed in injuries to the shoulder, knee, or hand.
106. **Cricothyroidotomy**: Emergency surgical procedure involving an incision through the skin and cricothyroid membrane to establish an airway, used in cases of upper airway obstruction.
107. **Partial Nephrectomy**: Surgical removal of a portion of a kidney, preserving the remaining healthy tissue, often done to treat kidney cancer.

108. **Tympanoplasty**: Surgical reconstruction of the eardrum or middle ear bones, commonly performed to restore hearing in cases of chronic ear infections or trauma.
109. **Stapedectomy**: Surgical removal or repair of the stapes bone in the middle ear, often used to treat hearing loss caused by otosclerosis.
110. **Percutaneous Transhepatic Cholangiography (PTC)**: A diagnostic procedure involving the insertion of a needle through the liver to visualize the biliary system, often used to diagnose and treat bile duct problems.
111. **Pulmonary Lobectomy**: Surgical removal of one of the lobes of the lung, often performed to treat lung cancer or other lung diseases.
112. **Oophoropexy**: Surgical fixation of an ovary, typically done to treat ovarian torsion (twisting) and preserve ovarian function.
113. **Laryngectomy**: Surgical removal of the larynx (voice box), often performed to treat laryngeal cancer, after which the patient breathes through a stoma (opening) in the neck.
114. **Femoral Popliteal Bypass**: A surgical procedure to create a new blood vessel pathway around a blocked femoral or popliteal artery, commonly done to treat peripheral arterial disease.
115. **Lithotripsy**: Non-invasive surgical procedure that uses shock waves to break up kidney stones or gallstones, allowing them to pass out of the body more easily.
116. **Cystectomy with Ileal Conduit**: Surgical removal of the bladder, with the creation of a urinary diversion using a piece of the small intestine (ileum) to form a conduit for urine to exit the body through a stoma.
117. **Axillary Lymph Node Dissection**: Surgical removal of lymph nodes in the armpit area, often performed to assess the spread of breast cancer.
118. **Bariatric Surgery**: Various surgical procedures, such as gastric bypass or sleeve gastrectomy, are performed to help individuals with obesity lose weight and improve related health conditions.
119. **Hemilaminectomy**: Surgical removal of one side of a vertebral bone (lamina), often done to decompress the spinal cord or nerves in cases of spinal stenosis or herniated discs.

120. **Vitrectomy**: A surgical procedure to remove the vitreous gel from the eye, often performed to treat conditions like retinal detachment or diabetic retinopathy.
121. **Esophageal Dilation**: A surgical procedure to stretch or dilate a narrowed or blocked portion of the esophagus, often due to conditions like strictures or achalasia.
122. **Cervical Laminoplasty**: A surgical procedure to create more space in the spinal canal by expanding the cervical vertebrae, commonly done to treat spinal cord compression.
123. **Pterygium Excision**: Surgical removal of a growth on the eye's surface, often performed when a pterygium (a pink, fleshy tissue) starts to affect vision.
124. **Inguinal Hernia Repair**: Surgical procedure to correct a hernia in the groin area, where abdominal tissue protrudes through a weak spot in the abdominal wall muscles.
125. **Transurethral Resection of the Prostate (TURP)**: Surgical procedure to treat benign prostatic hyperplasia (enlarged prostate) by removing portions of the prostate gland through the urethra.
126. **Bunionectomy**: Surgical removal of a bunion, a bony bump that forms at the base of the big toe, often causing pain and discomfort.
127. **Hip Arthroscopy**: Minimally invasive surgical procedure to diagnose and treat problems in the hip joint using a small camera and specialized instruments.
128. **Excisional Biopsy**: Surgical removal of an entire lump or suspicious area for examination, often performed to diagnose or rule out cancer.
129. **Scleral Buckling**: A surgical technique to repair a retinal detachment by indenting the wall of the eye (sclera) with a silicone band or buckle.
130. **Lobectomy (Liver)**: Surgical removal of a lobe of the liver, typically performed to treat liver tumors or liver disease.
131. **Umbilical Hernia Repair**: A surgical procedure to repair a hernia that occurs at or near the belly button, where abdominal tissue protrudes through a weak spot in the abdominal wall.
132. **Cricopharyngeal Myotomy**: A surgical procedure to treat difficulty swallowing (dysphagia) by cutting the cricopharyngeal muscle at the top of the esophagus.

133. **Pilonidal Cystectomy**: Surgical removal of a pilonidal cyst, a small sac that forms under the skin at the base of the spine, often requiring drainage or excision.
134. **Thyroglossal Duct Cyst Excision**: Surgical removal of a cyst or mass that forms from remnants of the thyroglossal duct, a structure present during embryonic development.
135. **Ulnar Nerve Transposition**: A surgical procedure to move the ulnar nerve from behind the elbow to the front, often done to relieve pressure or pain associated with cubital tunnel syndrome.
136. **Thoracoscopic Sympathectomy**: Minimally invasive surgery to treat hyperhidrosis (excessive sweating) by cutting or clamping the sympathetic nerves in the chest.
137. **Ganglion Cyst Removal**: A surgical procedure to remove a ganglion cyst, a non-cancerous lump that often forms near joints or tendons, causing discomfort.
138. **Ventriculostomy**: A surgical procedure to create an opening in the brain's ventricles to drain cerebrospinal fluid, often used to relieve increased intracranial pressure.
139. **Ureteral Stent Placement**: Surgical placement of a small tube (stent) in the ureter to ensure proper drainage of urine from the kidney to the bladder, commonly used after kidney stone removal or in cases of ureteral obstruction.
140. **Tonsillectomy** and **Adenoidectomy**: Surgical removal of the tonsils and adenoids, often performed to treat recurrent tonsillitis or breathing difficulties due to enlarged adenoids.
141. **Laparoscopic Nissen Fundoplication**: Minimally invasive procedure to treat gastroesophageal reflux disease (GERD) by wrapping the top of the stomach around the lower esophagus to prevent acid reflux.
142. **Meningioma Resection**: Surgical removal of a meningioma, a type of tumor that forms in the meninges, the layers of tissue covering the brain and spinal cord.
143. **Thyroid Lobectomy**: Surgical removal of one lobe of the thyroid gland, often done to treat thyroid nodules or thyroid cancer confined to one lobe.

144. **Cholecystojejunostomy**: Surgical creation of an opening between the gallbladder and the jejunum (part of the small intestine), often performed to bypass an obstruction in the common bile duct.
145. **Bilateral Salpingo-Oophorectomy**: Surgical removal of both fallopian tubes and ovaries, commonly done as a preventive measure for women at high risk of ovarian or breast cancer.
146. **Excisional Skin Biopsy**: Surgical removal of a suspicious skin lesion or mole for examination, often used to diagnose or rule out skin cancer.
147. **Spinal Fusion**: A surgical procedure to join two or more vertebrae in the spine, often done to stabilize the spine, treat spinal deformities, or alleviate pain.
148. **Temporal Lobectomy**: Surgical removal of the temporal lobe of the brain, usually performed to treat seizures that originate in this area (temporal lobe epilepsy).
149. **Cubital Tunnel Release**: A surgical procedure to relieve pressure on the ulnar nerve at the elbow, commonly done to treat cubital tunnel syndrome, a condition similar to carpal tunnel syndrome but involving the elbow.
150. **Partial Glossectomy**: Surgical removal of a portion of the tongue, often performed to treat oral cancer while preserving speech and swallowing functions.
151. **Pleurodesis**: Surgical procedure to create adhesions between the pleura (membranes surrounding the lungs) to prevent recurrent pleural effusion (accumulation of fluid around the lungs).
152. **Percutaneous Nephrolithotomy**: Minimally invasive procedure to remove kidney stones through a small incision in the back, typically done for large or complex stones.
153. **Laryngoscopy**: A medical procedure to visualize the larynx (voice box) using a laryngoscope, often used to diagnose voice or breathing problems.
154. **Vagotomy**: A surgical procedure to cut the vagus nerve, often performed to reduce stomach acid production in cases of ulcers or severe gastroesophageal reflux disease (GERD).
155. **Turbinectomy**: Surgical removal or reduction of nasal turbinates (bony structures inside the nose), often done to improve airflow in cases of nasal obstruction.

156. **Endovascular Aneurysm Repair (EVAR)**: Minimally invasive procedure to treat an aortic aneurysm by placing a stent graft inside the weakened vessel, preventing rupture.
157. **Cervical Cerclage**: A surgical procedure to sew the cervix closed during pregnancy to prevent premature birth, often done in cases of cervical insufficiency.
158. **Laser Lithotripsy**: A medical procedure using laser energy to break up kidney stones, allowing them to pass more easily or be removed through other means.
159. **Umbilical Herniorrhaphy**: Surgical repair of an umbilical hernia, a bulge near the navel caused by a weakness in the abdominal wall.
160. **Inguinal Lymph Node Dissection**: Surgical removal of lymph nodes in the groin area, often performed to assess the spread of cancer or treat lymphatic system disorders.
161. **Laparoscopic Appendectomy**: Minimally invasive surgical removal of the appendix, often performed in cases of appendicitis.
162. **Bilateral Mastectomy**: Surgical removal of both breasts, often done as a preventive measure or as a treatment for breast cancer.
163. **Trabeculectomy**: A surgical procedure to create a drainage opening in the eye for treating glaucoma and reducing intraocular pressure.
164. **Pancreaticoduodenectomy (Whipple Procedure)**: Surgical removal of the head of the pancreas, the duodenum, and other surrounding structures, often used to treat pancreatic cancer.
165. **Partial Hepatectomy**: Surgical removal of a portion of the liver, typically done to treat liver tumors or liver diseases.

Abdominal Aortic Aneurysm (AAA)

Definition: Abnormal bulging or ballooning of the abdominal aorta, a major blood vessel.

Pathophysiology: Weakening of the aortic wall, often due to atherosclerosis.

Signs and Symptoms: Often asymptomatic; pulsating abdominal mass, abdominal or back pain if symptomatic.

Causes/Risk Factors: Smoking, hypertension, atherosclerosis, genetic factors.

Medical Management: Blood pressure control, surveillance for growth.

Surgical Management: Endovascular stent grafting or open surgical repair for larger aneurysms.

Prognosis: The risk of rupture is high in untreated cases; elective surgery improves outcomes.

Interesting Fact: AAA can be life-threatening if it ruptures, causing massive internal bleeding.

Abdominal Compartment Syndrome

Definition: Increased intra-abdominal pressure leading to organ dysfunction.

Pathophysiology: Elevated pressure within the abdominal cavity, compromising blood flow to organs.

Signs and Symptoms: Abdominal distension, respiratory distress, elevated intra-abdominal pressure.

Causes/Risk Factors: Abdominal trauma, severe burns, massive fluid resuscitation.

Medical Management: Decompressive laparotomy, and supportive care in the intensive care unit.

Surgical Management: Surgical decompression, temporary closure techniques.

Prognosis: Depends on the underlying cause and timely intervention; can be life-threatening if untreated.

Interesting Fact: Abdominal compartment syndrome can occur in critically ill patients and requires close monitoring for early detection.

Abdominal or Retroperitoneal Sarcoma

Definition: Abdominal or retroperitoneal sarcomas are rare tumors that arise from soft tissues in the abdominal cavity or retroperitoneal space.

Pathophysiology: Genetic mutations in mesenchymal cells lead to uncontrolled growth, forming sarcomas.

Signs and Symptoms: Abdominal pain, a palpable mass, changes in bowel habits, and in advanced cases, symptoms due to compression of nearby structures.

Causes/Risk Factors: Genetic predisposition, certain inherited syndromes, and exposure to radiation might increase the risk.

Medical Management: Chemotherapy, radiation therapy, and targeted therapy to shrink the tumor before surgery. Surgical resection of the tumor, often involving surrounding tissues.

Surgical Management: Wide surgical excision to remove the tumor along with surrounding tissues to achieve clear margins.

Prognosis: Prognosis varies based on the tumor type, size, location, and stage at diagnosis. Complete surgical removal offers the best chance of cure.

Interesting Fact: Sarcomas can develop in various soft tissues, making their diagnosis and treatment complex.

Abdominal Trauma

Definition: Abdominal trauma refers to injuries to the abdomen and its contents, often resulting from accidents, falls, or assaults.

Pathophysiology: Blunt or penetrating force causes damage to internal organs, blood vessels, or abdominal wall structures.

Signs and Symptoms: Abdominal pain, tenderness, distension, bruising, signs of shock, and in severe cases, evisceration.

Causes/Risk Factors: Accidents, falls, sports injuries, or physical assaults.

Medical Management: Stabilization, pain control, and diagnostic imaging (CT scans) to assess internal injuries.

Surgical Management: Surgical exploration to assess and repair internal injuries, control bleeding, and prevent infection.

Prognosis: Prognosis varies widely based on the nature and extent of the injury. Prompt medical and surgical intervention can improve outcomes.

Interesting Fact: Abdominal trauma can involve injuries to multiple organs, requiring a multidisciplinary approach for effective treatment.

Abdominal Wall Hernia

Definition: Protrusion of abdominal organs through a weak spot in the abdominal wall muscles.

Pathophysiology: Weakness in the abdominal wall, allowing abdominal contents to herniate.

Signs and Symptoms: Visible bulge, pain, discomfort, especially during lifting or straining.

Causes/Risk Factors: Weak abdominal muscles, previous surgery, obesity, pregnancy.

Medical Management: Supportive garments, lifestyle modifications, avoiding heavy lifting.

Surgical Management: Hernia repair through open or laparoscopic surgery.
Prognosis: Excellent with surgical intervention; risk of recurrence if not repaired.

Interesting Fact: Abdominal wall hernias can occur in various locations, including inguinal, femoral, umbilical, and incisional hernias.

Accessory Spleen Removal

Definition: Accessory spleens are small, additional spleen tissue masses that may cause discomfort or complications, necessitating their removal.

Pathophysiology: Accessory spleens result from embryonic remnants and are usually harmless. However, if they cause symptoms or complications, surgical removal may be required.

Signs and Symptoms: Pain or discomfort in the left upper abdomen, especially if the accessory spleen compresses nearby organs or experiences torsion.

Causes/Risk Factors: Congenital factors lead to the presence of accessory spleens. Most are asymptomatic, but complications can arise in some cases.

Medical Management: Symptomatic management, imaging studies, and evaluation to confirm the presence and location of the accessory spleen.

Surgical Management: Accessory spleen removal (splenectomy) is performed to excise the additional spleen tissue, relieving symptoms and preventing complications.

Prognosis: Removal of accessory spleens typically resolves symptoms, providing relief to affected individuals.

Interesting Fact: Accessory spleens are a normal variation in human anatomy, occurring in approximately 10-30% of individuals. Surgical removal is only necessary if they cause problems.

Achalasia

Definition: Neurological disorder affecting the esophagus, leading to difficulty swallowing and impaired esophageal motility.

Pathophysiology: Loss of nerve cells in the esophagus, leading to decreased peristalsis and impaired lower esophageal sphincter relaxation.

Signs and Symptoms: Dysphagia (difficulty swallowing), regurgitation, chest pain, weight loss.

Causes/Risk Factors: Unknown; possibly autoimmune or genetic factors.

Medical Management: Calcium channel blockers, nitrates, botulinum toxin injections, pneumatic dilation.

Surgical Management: Heller myotomy (a surgical division of the esophageal muscle), fundoplication if reflux is present.

Prognosis: Generally good with appropriate interventions; symptoms can be managed effectively.

Interesting Fact: Achalasia is a rare disorder and can be challenging to diagnose due to its similarity to other esophageal conditions.

Acute Cholecystitis

Definition: Inflammation of the gallbladder, often due to gallstones blocking the cystic duct.

Pathophysiology: Blockage of the cystic duct, leading to gallbladder inflammation and sometimes infection.

Signs and Symptoms: Severe right upper abdominal pain, fever, nausea, vomiting, positive Murphy's sign.

Causes/Risk Factors: Gallstones, obesity, rapid weight loss, pregnancy.

Medical Management: Fasting, intravenous fluids, antibiotics, pain management.

Surgical Management: Cholecystectomy (removal of the gallbladder) during the acute phase or after resolution.

Prognosis: Good with timely intervention; can lead to complications like gangrene or perforation if untreated.

Interesting Fact: Acute cholecystitis is a common reason for hospitalization and surgery, often occurring due to gallstone obstruction.

Acute Perforated Peptic Ulcer

Definition: A peptic ulcer that has eroded through the wall of the stomach or duodenum, leading to leakage of digestive juices into the abdominal cavity.

Pathophysiology: Chronic inflammation weakens the ulcer site, which can perforate due to increased pressure from gastric acids.

Signs and Symptoms: Sudden, severe abdominal pain, guarding, rigidity, rebound tenderness, and signs of shock.

Causes/Risk Factors: Helicobacter pylori infection, NSAID use, smoking, and alcohol consumption.

Medical Management: Intravenous fluids, antibiotics, and acid-suppressing medications.

Surgical Management: Emergency laparotomy to repair the perforation and, in some cases, remove part of the ulcer.

Prognosis: Prognosis depends on the extent of the perforation and timely surgical intervention. Mortality rates are higher in older adults.

Interesting Fact: Perforated peptic ulcers are surgical emergencies with a high risk of complications if not promptly treated.

Adenoid Cystic Carcinoma

Definition: Slow-growing malignant tumor arising from glandular tissues, often involving salivary glands.

Pathophysiology: Uncontrolled cell growth in glandular tissues, forming a characteristic cribriform pattern.

Signs and Symptoms: Palpable mass, pain, cranial nerve involvement if near the head and neck area.

Causes/Risk Factors: Unknown; genetic mutations may play a role.

Medical Management: Chemotherapy, radiation therapy.

Surgical Management: Wide local excision, sometimes involving nerve resection.

Prognosis: Variable; tends to recur locally after excision.

Interesting Fact: Adenoid cystic carcinoma is known for its indolent nature and prolonged clinical course, often requiring long-term management.

Adrenal Adenoma

Definition: Adrenal adenoma is a benign tumor originating in the adrenal glands.

Pathophysiology: Adrenal adenomas are usually non-functional, but some can produce hormones, leading to various disorders (Cushing's syndrome, Conn's syndrome).

Signs and Symptoms: Often asymptomatic. If functional, symptoms depend on the hormones produced (e.g., hypertension in Conn's syndrome, weight gain in Cushing's syndrome).

Causes/Risk Factors: The exact cause is unknown. Certain genetic syndromes might predispose individuals to adrenal adenomas.

Medical Management: Observation for non-functional adenomas. Functional adenomas may require medications to control hormone production.

Surgical Management: Surgical removal (adrenalectomy) if the tumor is functional, causing symptoms, or if there's suspicion of malignancy.

Prognosis: The prognosis for benign adrenal adenomas is excellent after surgical removal.

Interesting Fact: Many adrenal adenomas are discovered incidentally during imaging for unrelated issues.

Adrenal Hemorrhage

Definition: Adrenal hemorrhage is bleeding into the adrenal glands, often caused by trauma, surgery, or certain medical conditions.

Pathophysiology: Disruption of blood vessels in the adrenal glands, leading to bleeding.

Signs and Symptoms: Abdominal or flank pain, low blood pressure, rapid heartbeat, and dizziness.

Causes/Risk Factors: Trauma, surgery, sepsis, or underlying bleeding disorders.

Medical Management: Stabilizing the patient, addressing the underlying cause, and managing symptoms.

Surgical Management: Surgery might be necessary in severe cases to control bleeding and remove damaged tissue.

Prognosis: Prognosis depends on the underlying cause and the extent of adrenal damage. Timely intervention is crucial.

Interesting Fact: Adrenal hemorrhage can present as a medical emergency, requiring swift diagnosis and intervention to prevent complications.

Adrenal Incidentaloma

Definition: Unintentionally discovered adrenal mass, often found during imaging studies for unrelated issues.

Pathophysiology: Benign or malignant growth in the adrenal gland.

Signs and Symptoms: Often asymptomatic; may cause hormonal imbalances if functional.

Causes/Risk Factors: Usually sporadic; some cases are related to genetic syndromes.

Medical Management: Hormonal evaluation, imaging surveillance.

Surgical Management: Surgery for functional or suspicious masses.

Prognosis: Good for benign masses; variable for malignant tumors.

Interesting Fact: With advances in imaging technology, adrenal incidentalomas are increasingly detected, posing challenges in management decisions.

Adrenal Insufficiency (Addison's Disease)

Definition: A condition where the adrenal glands do not produce enough hormones, primarily cortisol and aldosterone.

Pathophysiology: Autoimmune destruction of adrenal glands, infections, or certain medications.

Signs and Symptoms: Fatigue, weight loss, low blood pressure, hyperpigmentation, salt cravings.

Causes/Risk Factors: Autoimmune disorders, infections (such as tuberculosis), adrenal gland disorders.

Medical Management: Hormone replacement therapy (corticosteroids and mineralocorticoids).

Surgical Management: Not applicable for primary adrenal insufficiency; may be necessary if caused by adrenal tumors.

Prognosis: Good with lifelong hormone replacement therapy; requires regular monitoring.

Interesting Fact: Addison's disease can present with nonspecific symptoms and often requires a high index of suspicion for diagnosis.

Adrenal Myelolipoma

Definition: Adrenal myelolipoma is a rare benign tumor composed of mature fat cells and bone marrow elements in the adrenal gland.

Pathophysiology: Development of a non-cancerous tumor containing fat and bone marrow tissue.

Signs and Symptoms: Often asymptomatic and discovered incidentally during imaging tests. Large tumors can cause abdominal pain.

Causes/Risk Factors: Not well understood, often considered a random occurrence.

Medical Management: Monitoring for growth, especially in asymptomatic cases.

Surgical Management: Adrenalectomy if the tumor is large, causing symptoms, or if it's difficult to distinguish from malignancy.

Prognosis: Prognosis is excellent after surgical removal. Adrenal myelolipomas are non-cancerous.

Interesting Fact: Adrenal myelolipomas are often found in imaging studies and are considered rare incidental findings.

Ameloblastoma

Definition: Benign but locally aggressive tumor originating from the odontogenic epithelium (in the jaw).

Pathophysiology: Uncontrolled cell growth in the jawbone.

Signs and Symptoms: Jaw swelling, pain, difficulty in chewing.

Causes/Risk Factors: Unknown; usually sporadic.

Medical Management: None; surgical intervention for removal.

Surgical Management: En bloc resection, sometimes involving reconstruction.

Prognosis: Good; recurrence is possible after incomplete excision.

Interesting Fact: Ameloblastomas are more common in the lower jaw and require complete surgical removal due to their locally aggressive nature.

Ampullary Cancer

Definition: Malignant tumor originating from the ampulla of Vater, where the common bile duct and pancreatic duct meet and enter the duodenum.

Pathophysiology: Uncontrolled cell growth in the ampullary region.

Signs and Symptoms: Jaundice, abdominal pain, weight loss, changes in stool color.

Causes/Risk Factors: Unknown; may be related to chronic inflammation or genetic factors.

Medical Management: Chemotherapy, radiation therapy.

Surgical Management: Whipple procedure (pancreaticoduodenectomy).

Prognosis: Generally better than other pancreatic cancers due to earlier symptoms and detection.

Interesting Fact: Ampullary cancer is a rare subtype of pancreatic cancer and often has a better prognosis than tumors originating from other parts of the pancreas.

Anal Abscess and Fistula

Definition: Collection of pus near the anus (abscess) or abnormal tunnel between the anus and skin surface (fistula).

Pathophysiology: Infection of anal glands leads to abscess formation; if not properly drained, it can result in a fistula.

Signs and Symptoms: Pain, swelling, redness, discharge, fever.

Causes/Risk Factors: Infection of anal glands.

Medical Management: Incision and drainage for abscess. Surgical intervention for fistula.

Surgical Management: Fistulotomy (opening and draining the fistula tract) or other specialized procedures.

Prognosis: Generally good with proper drainage and surgical management.

Interesting Fact: Anal fistulas often result from untreated or inadequately treated anal abscesses.

Anal Cancer

Definition: Malignant tumor in the tissues of the anus.

Pathophysiology: Uncontrolled cell growth in the anal tissues.

Signs and Symptoms: Anal pain, bleeding, changes in bowel habits, mass or lump.

Causes/Risk Factors: Human papillomavirus (HPV) infection, anal intercourse, smoking, immunosuppression.

Medical Management: Chemotherapy, radiation therapy, surgery.

Surgical Management: Surgical removal of the tumor (local excision or more extensive resection).

Prognosis: Depends on the stage; early detection improves outcomes.

Interesting Fact: Anal cancer is relatively rare compared to other gastrointestinal cancers.

Anal Fissures

Definition: Tear in the lining of the anal canal.

Pathophysiology: Trauma or injury to the anal mucosa leads to a tear.

Signs and Symptoms: Pain, bleeding, itching, especially during bowel movements.

Causes/Risk Factors: Constipation, diarrhea, childbirth, anal intercourse.

Medical Management: Dietary fiber, stool softeners, topical creams. Severe cases may require surgery.

Surgical Management: Lateral internal sphincterotomy to relax the anal sphincter muscles.

Prognosis: Generally good with appropriate management.

Interesting Fact: Chronic anal fissures can lead to a cycle of spasms and poor healing, requiring medical intervention.

Aortic Aneurysm

Definition: Abnormal bulge or ballooning of the aorta, the body's main artery.

Pathophysiology: Weakening of the artery wall, often due to atherosclerosis.

Signs and Symptoms: Often asymptomatic until rupture; back or abdominal pain in some cases.

Causes/Risk Factors: Smoking, hypertension, atherosclerosis, genetic factors.

Medical Management: Blood pressure control, surveillance for growth.

Surgical Management: Endovascular stent grafting or open surgical repair for larger aneurysms.

Prognosis: The risk of rupture is high in untreated cases.

Interesting Fact: Aortic aneurysms can occur in various parts of the aorta, including the abdominal and thoracic regions.

Aortoenteric Fistula

Definition: Abnormal connection between the aorta and the intestine, often leading to gastrointestinal bleeding.

Pathophysiology: Erosion or communication between the aorta and the intestine, allowing blood to enter the gastrointestinal tract.

Signs and Symptoms: Sudden, severe gastrointestinal bleeding, abdominal pain, signs of shock.

Causes/Risk Factors: Prior aortic surgery, aortic aneurysm, and prosthetic grafts.

Medical Management: Stabilizing the patient, blood transfusions, intravenous antibiotics.

Surgical Management: Surgical repair of the fistula, often requiring removal of infected graft material.

Prognosis: Guarded; aortoenteric fistulas are life-threatening and require immediate intervention.

Interesting Fact: Aortoenteric fistulas are rare but can lead to catastrophic bleeding and are often associated with prior vascular surgeries.

Aortoiliac Occlusive Disease

Definition: Aortoiliac occlusive disease refers to the blockage of the aorta or iliac arteries, often due to atherosclerosis.

Pathophysiology: Atherosclerotic plaques narrow or block the arteries, reducing blood flow to the lower extremities.

Signs and Symptoms: Claudication, cold extremities, absent or diminished pulses, and erectile dysfunction in men.

Causes/Risk Factors: Atherosclerosis, smoking, high blood pressure, and diabetes.

Medical Management: Lifestyle modifications, antiplatelet medications, and supervised exercise programs.

Surgical Management: Angioplasty, stent placement, or bypass surgery.

Prognosis: Prognosis depends on disease severity. Early intervention can improve symptoms and prevent complications.

Interesting Fact: Aortoiliac occlusive disease can significantly impact a person's quality of life, but appropriate interventions can often provide relief.

Appendiceal Abscess

Definition: Localized collection of pus around the appendix, often resulting from untreated appendicitis.

Pathophysiology: Infection of the appendix leading to abscess formation.

Signs and Symptoms: Right lower quadrant pain, fever, abdominal tenderness, palpable mass.

Causes/Risk Factors: Acute appendicitis left untreated, perforated appendix.

Medical Management: Intravenous antibiotics, percutaneous drainage of the abscess.

Surgical Management: Interval appendectomy after resolution of the abscess.

Prognosis: Good with appropriate medical and surgical management; can recur if underlying appendicitis is not treated.

Interesting Fact: Appendiceal abscess can present with symptoms similar to acute appendicitis but requires a different approach to management.

Appendiceal Carcinoid Tumor

Definition: Rare tumor originating from neuroendocrine cells in the appendix.

Pathophysiology: Uncontrolled growth of neuroendocrine cells.

Signs and Symptoms: Often asymptomatic; can cause abdominal pain, and appendicitis-like symptoms.

Causes/Risk Factors: Unknown; usually sporadic.

Medical Management: Observation for small, asymptomatic tumors; surgery for larger or symptomatic tumors.

Surgical Management: Appendectomy; right hemicolectomy in advanced cases.

Prognosis: Generally good for localized tumors; variable for metastatic disease.

Interesting Fact: Appendiceal carcinoid tumors are a subset of neuroendocrine tumors and have a relatively better prognosis compared to other carcinoid tumors.

Appendiceal Goblet Cell Carcinoma

Definition: Appendiceal goblet cell carcinoma is a rare and aggressive type of cancer that originates in the appendix. It is characterized by the presence of goblet-shaped cells in the tumor tissue.

Pathophysiology: The exact cause is unknown, but it is thought to develop from normal goblet cells in the appendix. Genetic mutations and chronic inflammation might contribute to its formation.

Signs and Symptoms: Abdominal pain, changes in bowel habits, unexplained weight loss, and sometimes, symptoms resembling appendicitis.

Causes/Risk Factors: There are no specific known causes. Risk factors might include a history of inflammatory conditions of the appendix.

Medical Management: Chemotherapy, targeted therapy, and immunotherapy to slow down the progression of the disease.

Surgical Management: Surgery to remove the tumor, often involving removal of the appendix and surrounding tissues (right hemicolectomy).

Prognosis: Prognosis is generally poor due to the aggressive nature of the cancer. Early detection and complete surgical resection can improve outcomes.

Interesting Fact: Appendiceal goblet cell carcinoma is rare, accounting for less than 1% of all appendix tumors.

Appendiceal Mucocele

Definition: Appendiceal mucocele is a descriptive term for the distension of the appendix due to the accumulation of mucoid or gelatinous substance.

Pathophysiology: It occurs when the appendix becomes obstructed, preventing normal drainage of mucous secretions. This can result from various causes, including tumors or inflammation.

Signs and Symptoms: Often asymptomatic. When symptoms occur, they include abdominal pain, bloating, and changes in bowel habits. In severe cases, it can lead to appendicitis-like symptoms.

Causes/Risk Factors: Obstruction of the appendix lumen, which can result from tumors, fecaliths, or scarring from previous infections.

Medical Management: Observation and monitoring for changes. Surgical intervention is often necessary to prevent complications.

Surgical Management: Surgical removal of the appendix (appendectomy) and, in some cases, surrounding tissues if a tumor is present.

Prognosis: Prognosis is generally excellent with early diagnosis and surgical removal. If left untreated, it can lead to complications such as rupture.

Interesting Fact: Appendiceal mucoceles are rare, accounting for about 0.2-0.3% of all appendectomy specimens.

Appendicitis

Definition: Inflammation of the appendix, a small tubular structure attached to the colon.

Pathophysiology: Obstruction leads to bacterial overgrowth, inflammation, and potentially, perforation.

Signs and Symptoms: Right lower quadrant pain, nausea, vomiting, fever, and anorexia.

Causes/Risk Factors: Obstruction due to fecaliths, lymphoid hyperplasia, or tumors.

Medical Management: IV antibiotics, pain control. Surgery (appendectomy) is curative.

Surgical Management: Laparoscopic or open appendectomy.

Prognosis: Generally excellent but can be serious if perforated.

Interesting Fact: The function of the appendix is still debated in medical science.

Arterial Embolism

Definition: Arterial embolism occurs when an embolus, often a blood clot, blocks an artery, leading to reduced blood flow to the affected organ or limb.

Pathophysiology: Blood clots, fat, air, or other debris can travel through the bloodstream and lodge in an artery.

Signs and Symptoms: Sudden pain, pallor, pulselessness, paralysis, and coldness in the affected limb or organ.

Causes/Risk Factors: Atrial fibrillation, arterial plaque, or clots from deep veins (in cases of DVT).

Medical Management: Anticoagulant therapy, thrombolysis, and embolectomy.

Surgical Management: Embolectomy to remove the embolus and restore blood flow.

Prognosis: Prognosis depends on the location and duration of arterial occlusion. Prompt treatment improves outcomes.

Interesting Fact: Arterial embolism is a medical emergency requiring immediate intervention to prevent tissue damage or loss of limb function.

Arteriovenous Fistula

Definition: Arteriovenous fistula is an abnormal connection between an artery and a vein, often created intentionally for hemodialysis access.

Pathophysiology: Direct communication between artery and vein disrupts normal blood flow patterns.

Signs and Symptoms: Swelling, pulsation, and increased blood flow at the site of the fistula.

Causes/Risk Factors: Often created surgically for hemodialysis, but can occur due to trauma or congenital anomalies.

Medical Management: Monitoring for complications like aneurysm formation or ischemia.

Surgical Management: Closure of the fistula if it leads to complications or is no longer needed.

Prognosis: Prognosis is good after successful closure. Complications like aneurysm rupture can occur in untreated cases.

Interesting Fact: Arteriovenous fistulas are the preferred method for long-term hemodialysis access due to lower infection rates and longer patency.

Bariatric Surgery

Definition: Bariatric surgery is a medical procedure performed to help people with severe obesity lose weight. It involves making changes to the digestive system to limit the amount of food that can be eaten and/or reduce the body's ability to absorb nutrients.

Physiology: Bariatric surgeries work by either restricting the size of the stomach (restrictive procedures) or altering the way food is digested by bypassing parts of the stomach and small intestine (malabsorptive procedures). These changes lead to reduced calorie intake and nutrient absorption.

Signs and Symptoms: Bariatric surgery is not a condition with specific signs and symptoms; rather, it aims to alleviate symptoms associated with obesity, such as high blood pressure, diabetes, sleep apnea, and joint pain.

Causes: Severe obesity, often defined as having a body mass index (BMI) over 40, or a BMI over 35 with obesity-related health issues, like diabetes or high blood pressure. Risk factors include genetics, poor diet, lack of physical activity, and certain medical conditions.

Medical Management: Before surgery, patients undergo thorough evaluations, including psychological assessments, to determine their suitability for the procedure. Medical management also involves counseling, dietary changes, and exercise programs.

Surgical Management: There are several types of bariatric surgery, including gastric bypass, sleeve gastrectomy, and adjustable gastric banding. Gastric bypass involves creating a small pouch from the stomach and connecting it directly to the small intestine. Sleeve gastrectomy removes a portion of the stomach, leaving a smaller sleeve-shaped stomach. Adjustable gastric banding involves placing an inflatable band around the upper part of the stomach to create a smaller pouch.

Prognosis: Bariatric surgery can lead to significant weight loss, often resulting in the improvement or resolution of obesity-related health conditions. However, success requires a long-term commitment to lifestyle changes, including a healthy diet and regular exercise.

Interesting Facts:
Bariatric surgery is considered the most effective way for severely obese individuals to lose weight and improve their health.
After surgery, patients often experience rapid weight loss in the first few months, followed by a slower, steady weight reduction.
Bariatric surgery is not a cosmetic procedure but a medical intervention that can significantly enhance the quality of life for individuals struggling with obesity and related health issues.

Adjustable Gastric Banding

Definition: Adjustable gastric banding involves placing an inflatable band around the upper part of the stomach, creating a small pouch. The band can be tightened or loosened over time to control food intake.

Physiology: The band creates a small upper pouch, limiting food intake and promoting a sense of fullness. Adjustments can be made to control the size of the opening between the pouch and the rest of the stomach.

Surgical Management: The surgeon places a band around the upper stomach, creating a small pouch. A tube connected to the band allows for adjustments, which can be made by injecting or removing saline solution.

Prognosis: Adjustable gastric banding can result in moderate weight loss. However, it requires regular adjustments and may have a higher risk of long-term complications compared to other procedures.

Interesting Fact: Unlike other bariatric surgeries, adjustable gastric banding is reversible. The band can be removed if necessary, restoring the stomach to its original state.

Bariatric Revision Surgery

Definition: Bariatric revision surgery, also known as bariatric reoperation, is performed on individuals who have undergone a previous weight loss surgery but did not achieve the desired results or experienced complications.

Pathophysiology: Revision surgery corrects or modifies the results of a previous bariatric procedure. This can involve converting one type of surgery to another or addressing complications from the initial surgery.

Surgical Management: The specific surgical approach depends on the nature of the revision needed. It may involve resizing the stomach, correcting malabsorptive techniques, or addressing complications like gastric leaks.

Prognosis: Revision surgery can lead to improved weight loss outcomes and resolution of complications from the initial procedure. However, it carries higher risks due to the altered anatomy from the previous surgery.

Interesting Fact: Bariatric revision surgery requires careful evaluation and planning, as the altered anatomy from the initial surgery makes subsequent procedures more challenging.

Biliopancreatic Diversion with Duodenal Switch (BPD/DS)

Definition: BPD/DS is a complex bariatric surgery that combines restrictive and malabsorptive techniques. It involves removing a portion of the stomach and rerouting the small intestine to limit both food intake and nutrient absorption.

Physiology: The surgery reduces the stomach size, limiting the amount of food that can be consumed. It also reroutes the small intestine, reducing the absorption of calories and nutrients.

Surgical Management: A portion of the stomach is removed to create a smaller pouch. The small intestine is then rerouted to bypass a significant portion, reducing nutrient absorption.

Prognosis: BPD/DS often results in substantial weight loss, making it one of the most effective procedures for long-term weight management. However, it requires careful nutritional monitoring due to reduced nutrient absorption.

Interesting Fact: BPD/DS is typically recommended for individuals with a high BMI or those with obesity-related health conditions, as it leads to significant and sustained weight loss.

Gastric Balloon (Intragastric Balloon) Surgery

Definition: Gastric balloon surgery involves placing a deflated balloon into the stomach, which is then inflated to reduce the available space for food. It is a non-surgical, temporary weight loss procedure.

Physiology: The inflated balloon occupies space in the stomach, creating a feeling of fullness even with small meals. This reduces calorie intake and aids in weight loss.

Surgical Management: A deflated silicone balloon is inserted through the mouth and into the stomach, where it is inflated with saline solution. The procedure is typically performed endoscopically.

Prognosis: Gastric balloon surgery can lead to moderate weight loss over several months. The balloon is usually removed after six months to a year.

Interesting Fact: Gastric balloons are suitable for individuals with a lower BMI who do not qualify for more invasive procedures. They are temporary and can serve as a jumpstart to weight loss.

Gastric Bypass Surgery

Definition: Gastric bypass surgery, also known as Roux-en-Y gastric bypass, involves creating a small pouch from the upper part of the stomach and connecting it directly to the small intestine. This bypasses a portion of the stomach and the first section of the small intestine.

Physiology: By limiting the stomach's size and bypassing part of the small intestine, gastric bypass reduces the amount of food a person can eat and decreases nutrient absorption, leading to weight loss.

Surgical Management: The surgeon staples the stomach to create a small pouch, then connects it to the small intestine, bypassing the remaining stomach and upper part of the small intestine.

Prognosis: Gastric bypass typically results in significant weight loss, with patients losing a substantial amount of excess body weight within the first year after surgery.

Interesting Fact: Gastric bypass surgery not only reduces the stomach's size but also alters the hormones in the digestive system, affecting hunger and metabolism.

Mini-Gastric Bypass Surgery

Definition: Mini-gastric bypass is a simplified version of the traditional gastric bypass surgery. It involves creating a long narrow tube of the stomach and connecting it to a loop of the small intestine.

Physiology: By reducing the stomach size and bypassing a portion of the small intestine, mini-gastric bypass restricts food intake and alters nutrient absorption, leading to weight loss.

Surgical Management: The surgeon creates a small pouch from the stomach and connects it to a loop of the small intestine. The rerouted intestine reduces the absorption of calories and nutrients.

Prognosis: Mini-gastric bypass surgery can result in significant weight loss and improvement in obesity-related health conditions.

Interesting Fact: Mini-gastric bypass is less complex than traditional gastric bypass and often has a shorter operating time and hospital stay.

SADI-S (Single Anastomosis Duodeno-Ileal Bypass with Sleeve Gastrectomy)

Definition: SADI-S is a combination of sleeve gastrectomy and a modified form of duodenal switch surgery. It involves removing a portion of the stomach and rerouting the small intestine.

Physiology: SADI-S combines the restriction of food intake (from sleeve gastrectomy) with reduced nutrient absorption (from the modified intestinal bypass), leading to weight loss.

Surgical Management: The procedure involves sleeve gastrectomy to reduce stomach size and rerouting the small intestine to bypass a portion of it, reducing calorie and nutrient absorption.

Prognosis: SADI-S can lead to significant weight loss and improvement in obesity-related health conditions, similar to traditional duodenal switch surgery.

Interesting Fact: SADI-S is considered a more straightforward modification of the traditional duodenal switch surgery, aiming to achieve similar outcomes with potentially reduced complication rates.

Sleeve Gastrectomy

Definition: Sleeve gastrectomy involves removing a large portion of the stomach, leaving a banana-shaped sleeve. This procedure restricts the amount of food the stomach can hold and reduces the production of hunger-inducing hormones.

Physiology: By reducing the stomach's size, sleeve gastrectomy limits the amount of food intake, leading to weight loss. It also affects hormones that regulate hunger and satiety.

Surgical Management: The surgeon removes a significant portion of the stomach, leaving a narrow tube or sleeve. The smaller stomach restricts food intake, helping with weight loss.

Prognosis: Sleeve gastrectomy results in substantial weight loss and often improves or resolves obesity-related health conditions.

Interesting Fact: Unlike gastric bypass, sleeve gastrectomy does not involve rerouting the intestines, making it a simpler procedure with fewer complications related to nutrient absorption.

Benign Prostatic Hyperplasia (BPH)

Definition: Enlargement of the prostate gland in aging men.

Pathophysiology: Hormonal changes lead to glandular and stromal proliferation.

Signs and Symptoms: Urinary frequency, urgency, difficulty starting and stopping urination.

Causes/Risk Factors: Aging, hormonal changes, family history.

Medical Management: Alpha-blockers, 5-alpha reductase inhibitors, minimally invasive procedures.

Surgical Management: Transurethral resection of the prostate (TURP) for significant symptoms.

Prognosis: Generally good with appropriate management.

Interesting Fact: BPH is a common condition affecting older men and can cause bothersome urinary symptoms.

Biliary Colic

Definition: Severe pain due to gallstones obstructing the cystic duct or common bile duct.

Pathophysiology: Gallstones block the flow of bile, causing distension and pain.

Signs and Symptoms: Intense, cramp-like right upper quadrant pain, nausea, vomiting.

Causes/Risk Factors: Gallstones, obesity, rapid weight loss, pregnancy.

Medical Management: Pain management, dietary modifications, addressing underlying gallstones.

Surgical Management: Cholecystectomy (removal of the gallbladder) for recurrent or severe cases.

Prognosis: Excellent after surgical intervention; recurrence is rare after gallbladder removal.

Interesting Fact: Biliary colic often occurs after a fatty meal and can be triggered by specific foods.

Biliary Tract Disorders

Definition: Conditions affecting the bile ducts, including cholangitis, biliary strictures, and choledocholithiasis (stones in the bile ducts).

Pathophysiology: Obstruction or inflammation of the bile ducts leads to various disorders.

Signs and Symptoms: Jaundice, abdominal pain, fever, itching.

Causes/Risk Factors: Gallstones, inflammation, tumors.

Medical Management: ERCP (endoscopic retrograde cholangiopancreatography) for stone removal, and antibiotics for infections.

Surgical Management: Surgical intervention for strictures or tumors, often involving resection or bypass procedures.

Prognosis: Variable, depending on the specific disorder and its complications.

Interesting Fact: Gallstones can travel from the gallbladder into the bile ducts, causing obstruction and various complications.

Bleeding Esophageal Varices

Definition: Enlarged, swollen veins in the esophagus that can rupture and cause severe bleeding.

Pathophysiology: Portal hypertension leads to the formation of varices, often in liver cirrhosis.

Signs and Symptoms: Vomiting blood, black tarry stools (melena), low blood pressure.

Causes/Risk Factors: Liver cirrhosis, portal vein thrombosis.

Medical Management: Medications to reduce portal pressure, endoscopic band ligation.

Surgical Management: Transjugular intrahepatic portosystemic shunt (TIPS), variceal ligation.

Prognosis: Guarded; risk of rebleeding is significant.

Interesting Fact: Bleeding esophageal varices can be life-threatening and require urgent medical attention.

Boerhaave Syndrome

Definition: Spontaneous rupture of the esophagus, often due to severe vomiting or retching.

Pathophysiology: Increased intraesophageal pressure leading to esophageal wall rupture.

Signs and Symptoms: Severe chest pain, subcutaneous emphysema, fever.

Causes/Risk Factors: Forceful vomiting, alcohol intoxication, eating disorders.

Medical Management: NPO (nothing by mouth), antibiotics, IV fluids.

Surgical Management: Surgical repair, and drainage of mediastinal fluid.

Prognosis: Guarded; early diagnosis and intervention are crucial.

Interesting Fact: Boerhaave syndrome is a medical emergency often associated with significant morbidity and mortality.

Bowel Perforation

Definition: Hole or tear in the wall of the intestine, leading to leakage of contents into the abdominal cavity.

Pathophysiology: Trauma, ulceration, diverticulitis, or other gastrointestinal diseases can cause perforation.

Signs and Symptoms: Sudden severe abdominal pain, fever, vomiting, shock.

Causes/Risk Factors: Inflammatory conditions, trauma, cancer, infections.

Medical Management: Intravenous antibiotics, supportive care.

Surgical Management: Surgical repair of the perforation, and removal of damaged intestine.

Prognosis: Depends on the extent of the perforation and timely surgical intervention.

Interesting Fact: Bowel perforation is a surgical emergency and requires immediate intervention to prevent severe complications.

Breast Cancer

Definition: Malignant tumor in the breast tissue.

Pathophysiology: Genetic mutations lead to uncontrolled cell growth in breast tissue.

Signs and Symptoms: Lump in breast, changes in breast size/shape, nipple discharge, skin changes.

Causes/Risk Factors: Family history, BRCA gene mutations, hormonal factors, radiation exposure.

Medical Management: Surgery (lumpectomy or mastectomy), chemotherapy, radiation therapy, hormone therapy.

Surgical Management: Lumpectomy (removal of the tumor) or mastectomy (removal of the breast) depending on the stage.

Prognosis: Varies by stage; early detection significantly improves outcomes.

Interesting Fact: Breast cancer can occur in men, although it is rare, accounting for less than 1% of all breast cancer cases.

Bronchiectasis

Definition: Bronchiectasis is a chronic lung condition characterized by abnormal widening and thickening of the bronchial tubes, leading to mucus buildup.

Pathophysiology: Recurrent infections or inflammatory conditions damage the bronchial walls, leading to dilation and impaired mucus clearance.

Signs and Symptoms: Chronic cough with sputum production, wheezing, chest pain, and recurrent respiratory infections.

Causes/Risk Factors: Infections (especially in childhood), cystic fibrosis, immunodeficiency disorders, and aspiration.

Medical Management: Antibiotics, airway clearance techniques, bronchodilators, and immunizations to prevent infections.

Surgical Management: Surgery is reserved for severe cases or when localized bronchiectasis leads to recurrent infections. Lobectomy or segmentectomy may be performed.

Prognosis: Prognosis varies based on the underlying cause and the extent of lung damage. With proper management, many individuals can lead normal lives.

Interesting Fact: Chronic infections and inflammation in bronchiectasis can lead to irreversible lung damage, emphasizing the importance of preventive measures.

Bronchopulmonary Dysplasia (BPD)

Definition: BPD is a chronic lung disease that affects premature infants who require mechanical ventilation and oxygen therapy shortly after birth.

Pathophysiology: Lung injury from mechanical ventilation and oxygen toxicity leads to impaired lung development and function.

Signs and Symptoms: Respiratory distress, fast breathing, retractions (chest sinking in with each breath), and need for oxygen therapy.

Causes/Risk Factors: Premature birth, low birth weight, respiratory distress syndrome (RDS), and prolonged mechanical ventilation.

Medical Management: Oxygen therapy, bronchodilators, diuretics, and respiratory support.

Surgical Management: In severe cases, lung transplantation may be considered.

Prognosis: Prognosis varies; many infants improve as they grow, but some may have long-term respiratory issues.

Interesting Fact: BPD is a significant concern in neonatal intensive care units and requires a delicate balance of providing necessary respiratory support while minimizing lung injury.

Bronchopulmonary Sequestration

Definition: Bronchopulmonary sequestration is a congenital malformation where lung tissue lacks normal communication with the tracheobronchial tree and receives its blood supply from systemic arteries.

Pathophysiology: Improper embryonic development leads to the formation of a non-functioning lung tissue mass.

Signs and Symptoms: Respiratory distress in infants, recurrent lung infections, and chest pain in older children or adults.

Causes/Risk Factors: Congenital anomaly; exact causes are not well understood.

Medical Management: Antibiotics for infections, imaging studies for diagnosis, and surveillance for growth.

Surgical Management: Surgical resection of the affected lung tissue.

Prognosis: Prognosis is excellent after surgical removal. Patients can lead normal lives without the affected tissue.

Interesting Fact: Bronchopulmonary sequestration can sometimes be asymptomatic, and the condition may be discovered incidentally during imaging for unrelated issues.

Carotid Artery Disease

Definition: Narrowing or blockage of the carotid arteries, leading to reduced blood flow to the brain.

Pathophysiology: Atherosclerosis, plaque buildup in the carotid arteries, causing stenosis.

Signs and Symptoms: Transient ischemic attacks (TIAs), speech difficulties, weakness on one side of the body, and visual disturbances.

Causes/Risk Factors: Hypertension, smoking, diabetes, high cholesterol, and aging.

Medical Management: Blood pressure control, antiplatelet medications, statins.

Surgical Management: Carotid endarterectomy (surgical removal of plaque) or carotid angioplasty with stenting.

Prognosis: Excellent with prompt intervention; reduces the risk of stroke.

Interesting Fact: Carotid artery disease is a leading cause of stroke, and interventions aim to prevent stroke occurrence.

Cecal Volvulus

Definition: Twisting of the cecum (first part of the large intestine) upon itself, leading to obstruction.

Pathophysiology: Cecal rotation around its mesentery, causing bowel obstruction.

Signs and Symptoms: Abdominal pain, distension, constipation, vomiting, tenderness in the right lower abdomen.

Causes/Risk Factors: Congenital anomalies, previous abdominal surgery, abnormal mobility of the cecum.

Medical Management: Nasogastric decompression, fluid resuscitation, addressing electrolyte imbalances.

Surgical Management: Cecopexy (fixation of the cecum to the abdominal wall), cecostomy tube placement, or partial colectomy in severe cases.

Prognosis: Good with prompt surgical intervention; can lead to bowel necrosis if untreated.

Interesting Fact: Cecal volvulus is a relatively rare condition but requires urgent surgical evaluation and intervention to prevent complications.

Celiac Artery Compression Syndrome (Median Arcuate Ligament Syndrome)

Definition: Celiac artery compression syndrome occurs when the celiac artery is compressed by the median arcuate ligament, leading to abdominal pain and digestive issues.

Pathophysiology: Anatomic compression of the celiac artery by the median arcuate ligament during breathing or abdominal movements.

Signs and Symptoms: Abdominal pain after eating, weight loss, and digestive disturbances.

Causes/Risk Factors: Anatomical variation, often seen in young women.

Medical Management: Dietary changes, pain management, and lifestyle modifications.

Surgical Management: Division of the median arcuate ligament to relieve arterial compression.

Prognosis: Prognosis is excellent after surgical intervention, providing relief from symptoms.

Interesting Fact: Celiac artery compression syndrome is often underdiagnosed due to its rare occurrence and can mimic other gastrointestinal disorders.

Chest Wall Tumors

Definition: Chest wall tumors are abnormal growths in the bones, muscles, or soft tissues of the chest wall.

Pathophysiology: Tumors can be benign or malignant, arising from various tissues in the chest wall.

Signs and Symptoms: Pain, swelling, visible mass, or changes in the skin overlying the tumor.

Causes/Risk Factors: Genetics, radiation exposure, or environmental factors in certain cases.

Medical Management: Biopsy, imaging studies, and multidisciplinary evaluation.

Surgical Management: Surgical resection, often requiring complex reconstruction of the chest wall.

Prognosis: Prognosis varies widely based on tumor type, size, and location. Early detection and complete resection improve outcomes.

Interesting Fact: Chest wall tumors, though relatively rare, can encompass a diverse range of conditions. One intriguing aspect is their potential to manifest as secondary growths (metastases) from cancers originating in other parts of the body. For instance, breast cancer can metastasize to the bones of the chest wall. The complexity of these cases often necessitates collaboration among different medical specialties, including oncologists, radiologists, and surgeons, to ensure comprehensive evaluation and personalized treatment plans. Advances in imaging technologies and surgical techniques have significantly improved the precision of resections, leading to better outcomes and enhanced quality of life for affected individuals.

Cholangiocarcinoma

Definition: Malignant tumor arising from the cells lining the bile ducts inside and outside the liver.

Pathophysiology: Uncontrolled cell growth in the bile ducts, often associated with chronic inflammation.

Signs and Symptoms: Jaundice, abdominal pain, unexplained weight loss, itching, clay-colored stools.

Causes/Risk Factors: Primary sclerosing cholangitis, liver fluke infection, chronic biliary inflammation.

Medical Management: Chemotherapy, radiation therapy, targeted therapy.

Surgical Management: Surgical resection of the tumor, often combined with liver transplantation in some cases.

Prognosis: Poor; often diagnosed at an advanced stage, leading to limited treatment options.

Interesting Fact: Cholangiocarcinoma is a rare cancer but has a high mortality rate due to late-stage diagnosis and limited treatment options.

Cholecystitis

Definition: Inflammation of the gallbladder, often due to gallstones obstructing the cystic duct.

Pathophysiology: Gallstones block the flow of bile, leading to inflammation and infection.

Signs and Symptoms: Right upper quadrant pain, fever, nausea, vomiting, positive Murphy's sign.

Causes/Risk Factors: Gallstones, obesity, rapid weight loss.

Medical Management: NPO (nothing by mouth), IV fluids, antibiotics. Cholecystectomy for recurrent cases.

Surgical Management: Laparoscopic cholecystectomy is the standard procedure.

Prognosis: Excellent post-cholecystectomy.

Interesting Fact: Untreated cholecystitis can lead to serious complications, including gangrene and perforation.

Choledochal Cyst

Definition: Congenital cystic dilatation of the bile ducts, often involving the common bile duct.

Pathophysiology: Structural anomaly in the bile ducts, leading to cyst formation and bile flow obstruction.

Signs and Symptoms: Jaundice, abdominal pain, palpable mass, recurrent pancreatitis.

Causes/Risk Factors: Congenital anomaly, possibly genetic factors.

Medical Management: Symptomatic relief, antibiotics for cholangitis, addressing complications.

Surgical Management: Excision of the cyst and reconstruction of the biliary tract.

Prognosis: Good with timely surgical intervention; untreated cases can lead to complications like cholangitis and malignancy.

Interesting Fact: Choledochal cysts are a rare congenital anomaly and often require surgical correction to prevent complications.

Choledocholithiasis

Definition: Presence of gallstones in the common bile duct, leading to obstruction.

Pathophysiology: Gallstones migrate from the gallbladder to the common bile duct, causing obstruction and inflammation.

Signs and Symptoms: Jaundice, right upper quadrant pain, fever, nausea, vomiting.

Causes/Risk Factors: Gallstones, previous gallbladder surgery, biliary tract abnormalities.

Medical Management: ERCP with stone extraction, antibiotics, and pain management.

Surgical Management: Surgical removal of stones via choledochotomy during laparoscopic cholecystectomy.

Prognosis: Excellent with prompt intervention; can lead to complications if untreated.

Interesting Fact: Choledocholithiasis can cause serious complications such as pancreatitis if stones obstruct the pancreatic duct.

Chronic Mesenteric Ischemia

Definition: Gradual narrowing or blockage of the mesenteric arteries, leading to reduced blood flow to the intestines.

Pathophysiology: Atherosclerosis in mesenteric arteries causing reduced blood supply to the intestines.

Signs and Symptoms: Abdominal pain after eating (intestinal angina), weight loss, fear of eating.

Causes/Risk Factors: Atherosclerosis, smoking, diabetes, high blood pressure.

Medical Management: Lifestyle modifications, and medications to improve blood flow.

Surgical Management: Angioplasty and stenting, bypass surgery.

Prognosis: Good with timely intervention; can lead to complications like bowel infarction if untreated.

Interesting Fact: Chronic mesenteric ischemia often presents as postprandial abdominal pain and can be mistaken for other gastrointestinal disorders.

Chronic Pancreatitis

Definition: Persistent inflammation of the pancreas, leading to irreversible damage.

Pathophysiology: Long-term inflammation causing pancreatic tissue destruction.

Signs and Symptoms: Abdominal pain, weight loss, malabsorption, diabetes.

Causes/Risk Factors: Alcohol abuse, gallstones, genetic factors.

Medical Management: Pain management, pancreatic enzyme supplements, lifestyle modifications.

Surgical Management: Drainage procedures, sometimes total pancreatectomy in severe cases.

Prognosis: Variable; can be managed with appropriate interventions.

Interesting Fact: Chronic pancreatitis can significantly impact the quality of life due to chronic pain and nutritional issues.

Chylothorax

Definition: Chylothorax is the accumulation of chyle (lymphatic fluid containing fat) in the pleural cavity due to a leak in the thoracic duct.

Pathophysiology: Injury to the thoracic duct, often during surgery or trauma, leads to the leakage of chyle into the pleural space.

Signs and Symptoms: Shortness of breath, chest pain, cough, and milky-white pleural fluid.

Causes/Risk Factors: Trauma, surgery (especially cardiothoracic procedures), malignancies, or congenital malformations.

Medical Management: Dietary modifications (low-fat diet), drainage of pleural fluid, and octreotide therapy to reduce chyle production.

Surgical Management: Thoracic duct ligation or pleurodesis if conservative measures fail to stop the leakage.

Prognosis: The prognosis is good with appropriate management. Identifying and treating the underlying cause is essential for preventing recurrence.

Interesting Fact: Chylothorax can be a complication of major thoracic surgeries and requires careful postoperative management to prevent complications.

Chylous Ascites

Definition: Accumulation of milky lymphatic fluid in the abdominal cavity due to lymphatic vessel leakage.

Pathophysiology: Disruption or obstruction of lymphatic vessels, causing leakage of chyle (lymphatic fluid).

Signs and Symptoms: Abdominal distension, difficulty breathing, abdominal pain, nausea.

Causes/Risk Factors: Trauma, abdominal surgery, malignancy, congenital malformations.

Medical Management: Dietary modifications (low-fat diet), paracentesis, nutritional support.

Surgical Management: Lymphatic ligation, and shunting procedures to divert chyle away from the abdominal cavity.

Prognosis: Variable, depending on the underlying cause and effectiveness of treatment.

Interesting Fact: Chylous ascites can be challenging to manage and may require a multidisciplinary approach involving surgery, nutrition, and medical interventions.

Colon Cancer

Definition: Malignant growth in the colon or rectum.

Pathophysiology: Genetic mutations lead to uncontrolled cell growth in the colon lining.

Signs and Symptoms: Change in bowel habits, blood in stool, abdominal pain, weight loss.

Causes/Risk Factors: Family history, inflammatory bowel disease, age, diet high in red/processed meats.

Medical Management: Surgery, chemotherapy, radiation therapy.

Surgical Management: Colectomy (surgical removal of a portion of the colon) often with lymph node dissection.

Prognosis: Depends on the stage; early detection improves outcomes.

Interesting Fact: Colon cancer is one of the most preventable cancers through regular screenings like colonoscopies.

Colorectal Cancer

Definition: Malignant growth in the colon or rectum.

Pathophysiology: Genetic mutations lead to uncontrolled cell growth in the colon lining.

Signs and Symptoms: Change in bowel habits, blood in stool, abdominal pain, weight loss.

Causes/Risk Factors: Family history, inflammatory bowel disease, age, diet high in red/processed meats.

Medical Management: Surgery, chemotherapy, radiation therapy.

Surgical Management: Colectomy (partial or total removal of the colon) often with lymph node dissection.

Prognosis: Depends on the stage; early detection improves outcomes.

Interesting Fact: Colorectal cancer is the third most common cancer diagnosed in both men and women in the United States.

Colorectal Polyps

Definition: Colorectal polyps are abnormal growths in the colon or rectum that protrude from the inner lining of the intestinal wall.

Pathophysiology: Most polyps are benign, but some can develop into colorectal cancer over time. The exact cause is unclear but involves genetic and environmental factors.

Signs and Symptoms: Often asymptomatic. When symptoms occur, they might include blood in the stool, changes in bowel habits, abdominal pain, or anemia.

Causes/Risk Factors: Age, family history of colorectal polyps or cancer, inflammatory bowel disease, and certain genetic syndromes increase the risk.

Medical Management: Regular screenings (colonoscopies) to detect and remove polyps. Surveillance for individuals with a history of polyps.

Surgical Management: Surgical removal of large or cancerous polyps, or in cases where polyps are too numerous or difficult to remove endoscopically.

Prognosis: Prognosis is excellent if polyps are detected early and removed. Regular screenings are essential for prevention and early detection.

Interesting Fact: Colorectal polyps are common, and most are harmless. However, they are considered precancerous, making regular screenings crucial for cancer prevention.

Cystic Adventitial Disease

Definition: Rare vascular condition where a cyst forms within the outermost layer (adventitia) of an artery.

Pathophysiology: Cystic formation in the adventitial layer, often affecting peripheral arteries.

Signs and Symptoms: Claudication, limb pain, decreased pulse, aneurysm formation in severe cases.

Causes/Risk Factors: Unknown; often idiopathic.

Medical Management: None; surgical intervention for symptomatic or complicated cases.

Surgical Management: Cyst excision, vascular reconstruction if necessary.

Prognosis: Good with surgical intervention; recurrence is rare after complete excision.

Interesting Fact: Cystic adventitial disease is a rare cause of peripheral arterial disease and often affects young to middle-aged adults.

Deep Vein Thrombosis (DVT)

Definition: DVT is a blood clot that forms in a deep vein, usually in the legs.

Pathophysiology: Virchow's triad (venous stasis, endothelial injury, and hypercoagulability) contributes to clot formation.

Signs and Symptoms: Swelling, pain, warmth, and redness in the affected leg.

Causes/Risk Factors: Immobility, surgery, genetic factors (thrombophilia), and conditions like cancer.

Medical Management: Anticoagulants (blood thinners) to prevent clot extension and pulmonary embolism.

Surgical Management: Thrombectomy (clot removal) in severe cases.

Prognosis: Prognosis is good with timely intervention. However, untreated DVT can lead to pulmonary embolism, a life-threatening condition.

Interesting Fact: DVT can occur during long flights or immobility after surgery, emphasizing the importance of movement for prevention.

Desmoid Tumor

Definition: Aggressive fibrous tumor originating from musculoaponeurotic or mesenchymal tissues.

Pathophysiology: Uncontrolled cell growth in connective tissues.

Signs and Symptoms: Palpable mass, pain, limited range of motion if near joints.

Causes/Risk Factors: Genetic mutations, trauma.

Medical Management: Observation, anti-inflammatory medications, targeted therapy.

Surgical Management: Wide local excision; may be challenging due to proximity to vital structures.

Prognosis: Variable; tends to recur after excision.

Interesting Fact: Desmoid tumors are locally aggressive but do not metastasize to distant organs.

Diaphragmatic Hernia

Definition: Protrusion of abdominal organs into the chest cavity through a diaphragmatic defect.

Pathophysiology: Weakness or tear in the diaphragm, allowing abdominal contents to herniate.

Signs and Symptoms: Respiratory distress, abdominal pain, bowel sounds in the chest, cyanosis in infants.

Causes/Risk Factors: Congenital (in infants), traumatic (in adults).

Medical Management: Stabilization, respiratory support, addressing associated injuries.

Surgical Management: Hernia repair with diaphragmatic reconstruction.

Prognosis: Depends on the size and contents of the hernia; can cause respiratory compromise in severe cases.

Interesting Fact: Diaphragmatic hernias can be congenital (present at birth) or acquired due to trauma.

Diverticulitis

Definition: Inflammation or infection of diverticula (small pouches) in the colon wall.

Pathophysiology: Stool trapped in diverticula leads to inflammation or infection.

Signs and Symptoms: Left lower quadrant pain, fever, changes in bowel habits, nausea, vomiting.

Causes/Risk Factors: Low fiber diet, aging, obesity.

Medical Management: Antibiotics, clear liquid diet. Severe cases may require hospitalization.

Surgical Management: Surgery to remove the affected colon segment (resection) in complicated or recurrent cases.

Prognosis: Generally good with timely intervention.

Interesting Fact: Diverticulosis is common in older adults but not everyone with diverticula develops diverticulitis.

Diverticulosis

Definition: Presence of small pouches (diverticula) in the colon.

Pathophysiology: Weakness in the colon wall, often asymptomatic.

Signs and Symptoms: Often asymptomatic; diverticulitis can cause abdominal pain and changes in bowel habits.

Causes/Risk Factors: Aging, low-fiber diet.

Medical Management: High-fiber diet, symptomatic treatment.

Surgical Management: Surgery for complications like diverticulitis, abscess, or perforation.

Prognosis: Generally good, but complications can occur.

Interesting Fact: Diverticulosis is common, especially in older adults, and is often discovered incidentally during imaging studies.

Ectopic Pregnancy

Definition: Implantation of the embryo outside the uterus, often in the fallopian tubes.

Pathophysiology: Failure of the embryo to reach and implant in the uterus.

Signs and Symptoms: Abdominal pain, vaginal bleeding, shoulder pain (if rupture causes internal bleeding).

Causes/Risk Factors: Previous tubal surgery, pelvic inflammatory disease, smoking.

Medical Management: Methotrexate (in certain cases), monitoring for rupture.

Surgical Management: Laparoscopic salpingostomy or salpingectomy.

Prognosis: Good with early diagnosis and intervention; can be life-threatening if rupture occurs.

Interesting Fact: Ectopic pregnancies cannot proceed to full term and can cause severe bleeding if the fallopian tube ruptures.

Empyema

Definition: Empyema is a collection of pus in the pleural space, often occurring as a complication of pneumonia.

Pathophysiology: Bacterial infection in the lungs spreads to the pleural space, leading to an inflammatory response and pus accumulation.

Signs and Symptoms: Fever, pleuritic chest pain, cough with purulent or bloody sputum, and shortness of breath.

Causes/Risk Factors: Pneumonia, lung abscess, chest trauma, or a weakened immune system.

Medical Management: Antibiotics targeting the causative bacteria, thoracentesis for fluid drainage, and sometimes fibrinolytic therapy.

Surgical Management: Thoracic surgery for drainage, decortication (peeling off the infected pleural lining), or in severe cases, pleural space irrigation.

Prognosis: Prognosis varies based on the underlying cause and promptness of intervention. Timely drainage and appropriate antibiotics improve outcomes.

Interesting Fact: Empyema often requires a multidisciplinary approach involving pulmonologists, infectious disease specialists, and thoracic surgeons for optimal management.

Esophageal Cancer

Definition: Malignant tumor in the esophagus.

Pathophysiology: Genetic mutations due to chronic irritation (smoking, alcohol, acid reflux).

Signs and Symptoms: Dysphagia, weight loss, chest pain, coughing.

Causes/Risk Factors: Smoking, alcohol, chronic acid reflux (GERD).

Medical Management: Chemotherapy, radiation therapy, targeted therapy.

Surgical Management: Esophagectomy (removal of part or all of the esophagus) often with lymph node dissection.

Prognosis: Poor prognosis, especially in advanced stages.

Interesting Fact: Adenocarcinoma of the esophagus is more common in Western countries, while squamous cell carcinoma is prevalent in Eastern countries.

Esophageal Stricture

Definition: Esophageal stricture is the narrowing of the esophagus, often due to chronic gastroesophageal reflux disease (GERD) or esophageal cancer.

Pathophysiology: Chronic irritation or inflammation leads to the formation of scar tissue, causing narrowing of the esophageal lumen.

Signs and Symptoms: Difficulty swallowing (dysphagia), chest pain, regurgitation, and weight loss.

Causes/Risk Factors: GERD, esophageal cancer, prolonged use of a nasogastric tube, or ingestion of corrosive substances.

Medical Management: Acid-suppressing medications, endoscopic dilation, and dietary modifications.

Surgical Management: Esophageal dilation, esophageal stent placement, or in severe cases, esophagectomy with reconstruction.

Prognosis: Prognosis depends on the underlying cause and the extent of stricture. Early intervention often leads to better outcomes.

Interesting Fact: Severe esophageal strictures can significantly impact a person's quality of life, making swallowing difficult and uncomfortable.

Esophageal Varices

Definition: Dilated and swollen veins in the lower esophagus, often due to portal hypertension.

Pathophysiology: Increased pressure in the portal vein, leading to the development of collateral vessels in the esophagus.

Signs and Symptoms: Vomiting blood, black, tarry stools (melena), abdominal pain, signs of liver disease.

Causes/Risk Factors: Cirrhosis, portal vein thrombosis, alcoholic liver disease.

Medical Management: Medications to reduce portal pressure, endoscopic interventions (band ligation, sclerotherapy).

Surgical Management: Transjugular intrahepatic portosystemic shunt (TIPS), surgical shunting procedures in severe cases.

Prognosis: Guarded; risk of bleeding and mortality are high, especially with advanced liver disease.

Interesting Fact: Esophageal varices are a potentially life-threatening complication of liver disease and require close monitoring and intervention to prevent bleeding.

Fecal Incontinence

Definition: Inability to control bowel movements, leading to involuntary passage of stool.

Pathophysiology: Damage to the anal sphincter muscles or nerves.

Signs and Symptoms: Involuntary bowel movements, inability to control gas, social withdrawal.

Causes/Risk Factors: Childbirth trauma, anal surgery, nerve damage, aging.

Medical Management: Dietary modifications, medications, physical therapy.

Surgical Management: Sphincter repair, sacral nerve stimulation, colostomy in severe cases.

Prognosis: Variable, depending on the underlying cause and severity.

Interesting Fact: Fecal incontinence significantly impacts the quality of life and often goes unreported due to embarrassment.

Femoral Hernia

Definition: Hernia that protrudes through the femoral canal into the upper thigh.

Pathophysiology: Weakness in the femoral canal allows abdominal contents to herniate.

Signs and Symptoms: Groin bulge, discomfort, pain, especially during bending or lifting.

Causes/Risk Factors: Weakness in the femoral canal, obesity, pregnancy.

Medical Management: Supportive garments, lifestyle modifications, avoiding heavy lifting.

Surgical Management: Hernia repair through open or laparoscopic surgery.

Prognosis: Excellent with surgical intervention; risk of complications if left untreated.

Interesting Fact: Femoral hernias are more common in women and have a higher risk of incarceration compared to inguinal hernias.

Foreign Body Ingestion

Definition: Swallowing of objects or substances that are not intended for ingestion.

Pathophysiology: Ingested foreign bodies can cause obstruction, perforation, or other complications.

Signs and Symptoms: Throat discomfort, difficulty swallowing, abdominal pain, vomiting, bloody stools.

Causes/Risk Factors: Accidental ingestion, psychiatric conditions (pica), young children.

Medical Management: Observation, endoscopic removal.

Surgical Management: Surgery for complications such as perforation or severe obstruction.

Prognosis: Generally good with prompt removal; can be serious if complications occur.

Interesting Fact: Foreign body ingestion is common in children but can also occur in adults, especially those with psychiatric disorders.

Fournier's Gangrene

Definition: Rapidly progressing, life-threatening infection of the genital and perineal area.

Pathophysiology: Bacterial infection often originating from the skin or urinary tract, leading to necrotizing fasciitis.

Signs and Symptoms: Severe pain, swelling, crepitus (gas under the skin), fever, systemic toxicity.

Causes/Risk Factors: Diabetes, immunosuppression, local trauma, urogenital infections.

Medical Management: Intravenous antibiotics, aggressive fluid resuscitation, wound care.

Surgical Management: Surgical debridement of necrotic tissue, often requiring multiple procedures.

Prognosis: Poor without aggressive surgical intervention; high mortality rate.

Interesting Fact: Fournier's gangrene requires urgent and extensive surgical debridement to prevent the systemic spread of infection.

Gallbladder Cancer

Definition: Malignant tumor originating from the cells of the gallbladder.

Pathophysiology: Uncontrolled cell growth in the gallbladder lining, often associated with gallstones.

Signs and Symptoms: Jaundice, abdominal pain, unexplained weight loss, bloating.

Causes/Risk Factors: Gallstones, chronic inflammation of the gallbladder, porcelain gallbladder.

Medical Management: Chemotherapy, radiation therapy, targeted therapy.

Surgical Management: Cholecystectomy (removal of the gallbladder) with or without additional resection of nearby tissues.

Prognosis: Poor; often diagnosed at an advanced stage, leading to limited treatment options.

Interesting Fact: Gallbladder cancer is relatively rare but can be aggressive, often requiring a multidisciplinary approach for treatment.

Gallbladder Polyps

Definition: Small growths or lesions in the gallbladder wall.

Pathophysiology: Precise cause unknown; some polyps can progress to cancer.

Signs and Symptoms: Usually asymptomatic; discovered during imaging studies for other conditions.

Causes/Risk Factors: Genetic factors, inflammation, gallstones.

Medical Management: Monitoring with regular ultrasounds, and surgical removal if polyps are large or suspicious.

Surgical Management: Cholecystectomy (removal of the gallbladder) for large or suspicious polyps.

Prognosis: Generally good if detected early; risk of malignancy is low.

Interesting Fact: Most gallbladder polyps are benign, but surveillance is necessary due to the risk of cancerous transformation.

Gallstone Ileus

Definition: Bowel obstruction caused by the passage of a large gallstone into the small intestine.

Pathophysiology: Gallstone migrates from the gallbladder to the intestine, causing obstruction.

Signs and Symptoms: Abdominal pain, vomiting, distension, visible lump in the abdomen.

Causes/Risk Factors: Gallstones, gallbladder inflammation.

Medical Management: Intravenous fluids, pain management, decompression.

Surgical Management: Enterolithotomy (surgical removal of the gallstone) and possible cholecystectomy.

Prognosis: Good with surgical intervention; can lead to complications like bowel perforation if untreated.

Interesting Fact: Gallstone ileus is a rare cause of small bowel obstruction and requires a careful approach to management.

Gallstone Pancreatitis

Definition: Inflammation of the pancreas caused by gallstones obstructing the pancreatic duct.

Pathophysiology: Gallstones block the pancreatic duct, leading to autodigestion of the pancreas.

Signs and Symptoms: Severe upper abdominal pain, nausea, vomiting, and fever.

Causes/Risk Factors: Gallstones, obesity, rapid weight loss.

Medical Management: NPO (nothing by mouth), intravenous fluids, pain management, addressing underlying gallstones.

Surgical Management: ERCP (Endoscopic Retrograde Cholangiopancreatography) with sphincterotomy to remove stones, and cholecystectomy for recurrent cases.

Prognosis: Excellent with prompt medical or surgical intervention.

Interesting Fact: Gallstone pancreatitis is a common cause of acute pancreatitis.

Gallstones (Cholelithiasis) and Cholecystitis

Definition: Solid particles forming in the gallbladder or inflammation of the gallbladder due to stones.

Pathophysiology: Imbalance in bile components leading to stone formation; stones can obstruct bile flow, causing inflammation.

Signs and Symptoms: Severe right upper quadrant pain, nausea, vomiting, fever, and jaundice.

Causes/Risk Factors: High cholesterol, high bilirubin, obesity, pregnancy, rapid weight loss.

Medical Management: Dietary modifications, and medications to dissolve stones. Cholecystectomy is curative.

Surgical Management: Laparoscopic removal of the gallbladder.

Prognosis: Excellent post-cholecystectomy.

Interesting Fact: Gallstones are more common in females and can lead to complications like pancreatitis.

Gastric Cancer

Definition: Malignant tumor in the stomach lining.

Pathophysiology: Genetic mutations, often associated with chronic Helicobacter pylori infection.

Signs and Symptoms: Abdominal pain, nausea, weight loss, early satiety.

Causes/Risk Factors: H. pylori infection, smoking, family history, and certain dietary factors.

Medical Management: Chemotherapy, targeted therapy, immunotherapy.

Surgical Management: Partial or total gastrectomy (removal of part or all of the stomach) often with lymph node dissection.

Prognosis: Poor prognosis, especially in advanced stages.

Interesting Fact: The incidence of gastric cancer has declined over the years, possibly due to decreased rates of H. pylori infection and changes in diet.

Gastric Leiomyosarcoma

Definition: Gastric leiomyosarcoma is a malignant tumor that arises from smooth muscle cells in the stomach wall.

Pathophysiology: The tumor originates from the muscular layer of the stomach. Genetic mutations and factors triggering uncontrolled cell growth might contribute.

Signs and Symptoms: Abdominal pain, early satiety, weight loss, vomiting blood, anemia, and a palpable mass in the abdomen.

Causes/Risk Factors: Genetic predisposition and certain genetic syndromes might increase the risk. However, specific causes are not well understood.

Medical Management: Chemotherapy, radiation therapy, and targeted therapy to shrink the tumor before surgery. Post-surgery, adjuvant therapies may be used to prevent recurrence.

Surgical Management: Surgical removal of the tumor, often involving partial or total gastrectomy (removal of part or all of the stomach).

Prognosis: Prognosis varies based on the stage of the cancer at diagnosis. Complete surgical removal offers the best chance of long-term survival.

Interesting Fact: Leiomyosarcomas are rare tumors, and when they occur in the stomach, they pose a significant challenge in diagnosis and treatment.

Gastric Ulcer

Definition: Erosion or sore in the lining of the stomach, often due to Helicobacter pylori infection or NSAID use.

Pathophysiology: Imbalance between stomach acid and the protective mucous layer, leading to erosion of the stomach lining.

Signs and Symptoms: Burning stomach pain, bloating, nausea, vomiting, weight loss.

Causes/Risk Factors: Helicobacter pylori infection, NSAID use, excessive alcohol consumption, smoking.

Medical Management: Proton pump inhibitors, antibiotics for H. pylori eradication, avoiding irritants.

Surgical Management: Reserved for complications like perforation or bleeding; rarely required.

Prognosis: Excellent with appropriate medical management; recurrence is possible without lifestyle modifications.

Interesting Fact: Most gastric ulcers are associated with H. pylori infection and can be effectively treated with antibiotics.

Gastroesophageal Reflux Disease (GERD)

Definition: Chronic condition where stomach acid frequently flows back into the esophagus.

Pathophysiology: A weak lower esophageal sphincter allows stomach acid to reflux into the esophagus.

Signs and Symptoms: Heartburn, regurgitation, chest pain, difficulty swallowing, chronic cough.

Causes/Risk Factors: Obesity, hiatal hernia, pregnancy, smoking.

Medical Management: Antacids, proton pump inhibitors, lifestyle modifications.

Surgical Management: Fundoplication (surgical wrapping of the upper stomach around the lower esophagus) in severe cases.

Prognosis: Generally good with proper management; surgery provides long-term relief in refractory cases.

Interesting Fact: Chronic GERD can lead to complications like esophagitis, Barrett's esophagus, and esophageal cancer.

Gastrointestinal Bleeding

Definition: Bleeding that occurs in the gastrointestinal tract, often originating from the esophagus, stomach, or colon.

Pathophysiology: Various causes including ulcers, diverticulosis, esophageal varices, or cancer.

Signs and Symptoms: Melena (dark, tarry stools), hematemesis (vomiting blood), hematochezia (bright red or maroon-colored stools), weakness, dizziness.

Causes/Risk Factors: Peptic ulcers, gastritis, esophageal varices, colorectal polyps, Crohn's disease.

Medical Management: Endoscopy, blood transfusions, medications to stop bleeding.

Surgical Management: Surgery to repair or remove the bleeding source in severe cases.

Prognosis: Variable, depends on the underlying cause and timely intervention.

Interesting Fact: Gastrointestinal bleeding can be life-threatening and requires prompt medical attention.

Gastrointestinal Fistula

Definition: Abnormal connection between two parts of the gastrointestinal tract or between the GI tract and another organ.

Pathophysiology: Infection, inflammation, or surgical complications can lead to the formation of fistulas.

Signs and Symptoms: Drainage of fluid or stool from an opening on the skin, abdominal pain.

Causes/Risk Factors: Inflammatory bowel disease, cancer, surgical complications, trauma.

Medical Management: Antibiotics, nutritional support, wound care.

Surgical Management: Surgical closure or repair of the fistula.

Prognosis: Variable, depending on the underlying cause and extent of the fistula.

Interesting Fact: Gastrointestinal fistulas can significantly impact a patient's quality of life and often require complex surgical interventions.

Gastrointestinal or Abdominal Lymphoma

Definition: Gastrointestinal lymphoma refers to lymphomas that originate in the digestive system, including the stomach, small intestine, and colon.

Pathophysiology: Abnormal growth of lymphocytes in the gastrointestinal tract leads to the formation of lymphomas.

Signs and Symptoms: Abdominal pain, nausea, vomiting, changes in bowel habits, unexplained weight loss, and in some cases, gastrointestinal bleeding.

Causes/Risk Factors: Weakened immune system, certain infections (e.g., Helicobacter pylori in the stomach), and autoimmune conditions increase the risk.

Medical Management: Chemotherapy, radiation therapy, immunotherapy, and sometimes stem cell transplantation.

Surgical Management: Surgery might be necessary to remove obstructive masses or obtain tissue samples for diagnosis. Surgery is often combined with other treatments.

Prognosis: Prognosis varies based on the type of lymphoma, its location, and the stage at diagnosis.

Interesting Fact: Gastrointestinal lymphomas can be challenging to diagnose and differentiate from other gastrointestinal disorders.

Gastrointestinal Stromal Tumor (GIST)

Definition: Soft tissue sarcoma arising in the gastrointestinal tract.

Pathophysiology: Mutations in the c-KIT or PDGFRA genes leading to uncontrolled cell growth.

Signs and Symptoms: Abdominal pain, bleeding, mass in the abdomen.

Causes/Risk Factors: Genetic mutations.

Medical Management: Targeted therapy (imatinib), surgery for localized tumors.

Surgical Management: Surgical resection with clear margins.

Prognosis: Depends on size, location, and completeness of surgical resection.

Interesting Fact: GISTs can occur anywhere in the GI tract but are most common in the stomach.

Gastroparesis

Definition: Delayed emptying of the stomach, often due to impaired motility of the stomach muscles.

Pathophysiology: Damage to the vagus nerve or stomach muscles, leading to poor gastric emptying.

Signs and Symptoms: Nausea, vomiting, abdominal pain, bloating, early satiety.

Causes/Risk Factors: Diabetes, neurological disorders, surgery, certain medications.

Medical Management: Dietary modifications (small, frequent meals), medications to stimulate stomach emptying, and nutritional support.

Surgical Management: Gastric electrical stimulation, pyloroplasty (widening the pyloric opening), partial gastrectomy in severe cases.

Prognosis: Variable, depending on the underlying cause and response to treatment.

Interesting Fact: Gastroparesis can significantly impact the quality of life, leading to malnutrition and dehydration if not managed effectively.

Giant Cell Tumor of Bone

Definition: Locally aggressive tumor characterized by the presence of multinucleated giant cells.

Pathophysiology: Abnormal growth of stromal cells and giant cells.

Signs and Symptoms: Bone pain, swelling, limited range of motion.

Causes/Risk Factors: Unknown; usually sporadic.

Medical Management: Pain management, bisphosphonates, denosumab.

Surgical Management: Curettage and bone grafting, sometimes involving joint reconstruction.

Prognosis: Variable; tends to recur locally after excision.

Interesting Fact: Giant cell tumors of bone can cause significant bone destruction and tend to affect young adults.

Hemorrhoids

Definition: Swollen and inflamed veins in the rectum and anus.

Pathophysiology: Increased pressure in the veins of the rectum, causing them to swell and become painful.

Signs and Symptoms: Pain, bleeding during bowel movements, itching, discomfort.

Causes/Risk Factors: Straining during bowel movements, constipation, pregnancy, obesity.

Medical Management: Dietary modifications, topical treatments, lifestyle changes.

Surgical Management: Hemorrhoidectomy (surgical removal of hemorrhoids) for severe cases.

Prognosis: Generally good with appropriate management.

Interesting Fact: Hemorrhoids are a common condition, especially during pregnancy and in older adults.

Hepatic Abscess

Definition: Collection of pus in the liver, typically caused by bacterial infection.

Pathophysiology: Bacterial infection in the liver tissue, leading to abscess formation.

Signs and Symptoms: Right upper quadrant pain, fever, jaundice, weight loss.

Causes/Risk Factors: Biliary tract infection, abdominal trauma, immunosuppression.

Medical Management: Antibiotics, drainage of the abscess if necessary.

Surgical Management: Percutaneous drainage or open surgical drainage for large or complicated abscesses.

Prognosis: Good with prompt medical intervention; can be life-threatening if untreated.

Interesting Fact: Liver abscesses can be single or multiple and are often caused by bacterial spread from other parts of the body.

Hepatic Hemangioma

Definition: Benign tumor in the liver composed of tangled blood vessels.

Pathophysiology: Abnormal development of blood vessels in the liver.

Signs and Symptoms: Often asymptomatic; discovered incidentally during imaging studies.

Causes/Risk Factors: Unknown; may be congenital.

Medical Management: Observation, especially for small, asymptomatic hemangiomas.

Surgical Management: Surgical resection in symptomatic cases or if there's concern for rupture.

Prognosis: Excellent; benign nature, but intervention may be necessary if symptomatic.

Interesting Fact: Hepatic hemangiomas are the most common benign liver tumors and are usually discovered incidentally.

Hepatic Hydatid Cyst

Definition: Cystic growth caused by the larval stage of Echinococcus tapeworm, specifically in the liver.

Pathophysiology: Parasitic infection leading to cyst formation in the liver.

Signs and Symptoms: Often asymptomatic; can cause abdominal pain, jaundice, and hepatomegaly if large.

Causes/Risk Factors: Contact with infected animals, especially dogs.

Medical Management: Anti-parasitic medications.

Surgical Management: Cyst removal, sometimes requiring liver resection.

Prognosis: Good with surgical removal; recurrence possible if not completely excised.

Interesting Fact: Hepatic hydatid cysts are endemic in certain regions where livestock raising is common.

Hernias

Definition: Protrusion of an organ or tissue through a weak area in the abdominal wall.

Pathophysiology: Weakened abdominal wall combined with increased intra-abdominal pressure.

Signs and Symptoms: Visible lump, pain, and discomfort, especially during activities.

Causes/Risk Factors: Muscle weakness, congenital defects, heavy lifting, obesity, chronic coughing.

Medical Management: Supportive (truss). Surgical repair (herniorrhaphy) is definitive.

Surgical Management: Open or laparoscopic repair, often using mesh.

Prognosis: Generally good with low recurrence rates post-surgery.

Interesting Fact: Hernias can occur in various locations, including inguinal, femoral, umbilical, and hiatal regions.

Hiatal Hernia

Definition: Hernia where the upper part of the stomach protrudes into the chest through the diaphragm opening (hiatus).

Pathophysiology: Weakness in the diaphragm allows the stomach to push through the hiatus.

Signs and Symptoms: Heartburn, regurgitation, chest pain, difficulty swallowing.

Causes/Risk Factors: Weakness in the diaphragm, obesity, aging.

Medical Management: Antacids, proton pump inhibitors, lifestyle modifications.

Surgical Management: Hiatal hernia repair (fundoplication) is often combined with anti-reflux surgery.

Prognosis: Generally good, with surgery providing long-term relief in refractory cases.

Interesting Fact: Many people with hiatal hernias are asymptomatic and may not require treatment unless symptoms occur.

Hidradenitis Suppurativa

Definition: Chronic skin condition characterized by the formation of painful lumps under the skin, often in areas with sweat glands.

Pathophysiology: Inflammation of hair follicles and sweat glands, leading to abscess formation.

Signs and Symptoms: Painful lumps, abscesses, tunnels under the skin, scarring.

Causes/Risk Factors: Genetics, smoking, obesity, hormonal factors.

Medical Management: Antibiotics, anti-inflammatory medications, warm compresses.

Surgical Management: Incision and drainage of abscesses, wide excision in severe cases.

Prognosis: Chronic condition with periods of exacerbation and remission; requires long-term management.

Interesting Fact: Hidradenitis suppurativa can significantly impact the quality of life and often requires a multidisciplinary approach for management.

Hirschsprung's Disease

Definition: Congenital condition where certain portions of the colon lack nerve cells, leading to obstruction.

Pathophysiology: Absence of ganglion cells in the myenteric plexus of the affected colon segment.

Signs and Symptoms: Delayed passage of meconium in newborns, chronic constipation, abdominal distension.

Causes/Risk Factors: Genetic mutations, usually sporadic.

Medical Management: Rectal irrigations, dietary modifications, supportive care.

Surgical Management: Bowel resection, pull-through procedure.

Prognosis: Good with surgical correction; can have long-term bowel function issues.

Interesting Fact: Hirschsprung's disease is often diagnosed in infancy and requires surgical intervention to restore normal bowel function.

Hydrocele

Definition: Accumulation of fluid in the sac around the testes, causing scrotal swelling.

Pathophysiology: Imbalance between fluid production and absorption in the scrotum.

Signs and Symptoms: Scrotal swelling, discomfort, feeling of heaviness.

Causes/Risk Factors: Injury, infection, congenital defects.

Medical Management: Observation, aspiration (draining fluid with a needle), surgery for persistent cases.

Surgical Management: Hydrocelectomy (surgical removal of the hydrocele sac).

Prognosis: Excellent; recurrence is rare after successful surgery.

Interesting Fact: Hydroceles can occur at any age and may resolve spontaneously in infants but often require surgery in adults.

Hydronephrosis

Definition: Swelling of the kidney due to the backup of urine, often caused by an obstruction in the urinary tract.

Pathophysiology: Obstruction of urine flow, leading to dilation and swelling of the renal pelvis and calyces.

Signs and Symptoms: Flank pain, urinary urgency, frequency, hematuria (blood in urine).

Causes/Risk Factors: Kidney stones, tumors, urinary tract infections, congenital abnormalities.

Medical Management: Treating underlying causes, relieving obstruction, pain management.

Surgical Management: Ureteral stent placement, nephrostomy tube insertion, surgical correction of underlying causes.

Prognosis: Good with timely intervention; may lead to kidney damage if untreated.

Interesting Fact: Hydronephrosis can be a temporary condition if the underlying cause is identified and treated promptly.

Hyperparathyroidism-Jaw Tumor Syndrome

Definition: Hyperparathyroidism-jaw tumor syndrome is a rare genetic disorder characterized by the overactivity of parathyroid glands and the development of tumors in the jaw and other bones.

Pathophysiology: Genetic mutations cause overactivity of parathyroid glands and bone tumors.

Signs and Symptoms: High calcium levels, jaw tumors, kidney stones, and bone pain.

Causes/Risk Factors: Genetic mutations (CDC73 gene mutations).

Medical Management: Managing hypercalcemia, surgery to remove tumors and affected parathyroid glands.

Surgical Management: Parathyroidectomy and removal of jaw tumors, often involving complex procedures.

Prognosis: Prognosis depends on the extent of the disease and the success of surgical interventions.

Interesting Fact: Hyperparathyroidism-jaw tumor syndrome is extremely rare, with only a few documented cases worldwide.

Incarcerated Hernia

Definition: Hernia in which abdominal contents become trapped and cannot be pushed back into the abdomen.

Pathophysiology: Hernia opening narrows, trapping the contents.

Signs and Symptoms: Severe pain, swelling, redness, nausea, vomiting.

Causes/Risk Factors: Weakness in the abdominal wall, obesity, previous surgery.

Medical Management: IV fluids, pain management, and hernia reduction (if possible).

Surgical Management: Emergency hernia repair, sometimes involving resection of damaged tissue.

Prognosis: Good with prompt intervention; can be life-threatening if untreated.

Interesting Fact: Incarcerated hernias require urgent surgical attention to prevent complications such as strangulation and tissue necrosis.

Inflammatory Bowel Disease (IBD)

Definition: Chronic inflammation of the digestive tract, including Crohn's disease and ulcerative colitis.

Pathophysiology: Immune system dysfunction, genetic and environmental factors.

Signs and Symptoms: Diarrhea, abdominal pain, weight loss, fatigue.

Causes/Risk Factors: Genetic predisposition, environmental factors, dysregulated immune response.

Medical Management: Anti-inflammatory medications, immunosuppressants, biologics.

Surgical Management: Surgery for complications like strictures, fistulas, or intractable symptoms.

Prognosis: Variable, often relapsing and remitting.

Interesting Fact: IBD is more common in developed countries and among individuals of Ashkenazi Jewish descent.

Inguinal Hernia

Definition: Hernia that occurs in the inguinal canal, often in the groin area.

Pathophysiology: Weakness in the inguinal canal allows abdominal contents to protrude.

Signs and Symptoms: Bulge in the groin, discomfort, pain, especially when lifting.

Causes/Risk Factors: Muscle weakness, heavy lifting, chronic coughing, male gender.

Medical Management: Supportive measures (truss). Surgical repair (herniorrhaphy) is definitive.

Surgical Management: Repair using open or laparoscopic techniques, often involving mesh placement.

Prognosis: Generally good with low recurrence rates post-surgery.

Interesting Fact: Inguinal hernias are more common in men due to the natural weakness in the inguinal canal, a vestige from the testicular descent in fetal development.

Intestinal Ischemia

Definition: Inadequate blood supply to the intestines, leading to tissue damage and potential gangrene.

Pathophysiology: Occlusion or narrowing of mesenteric arteries or veins, causing inadequate blood supply to the intestines.

Signs and Symptoms: Severe abdominal pain, tenderness, vomiting, bloody stools, signs of shock.

Causes/Risk Factors: Atherosclerosis, embolism, thrombosis, mesenteric venous thrombosis.

Medical Management: Intravenous fluids, anticoagulants, addressing underlying causes.

Surgical Management: Revascularization procedures, bowel resection for necrotic tissue.

Prognosis: Variable, depending on the extent of ischemia and timely intervention.

Interesting Fact: Intestinal ischemia is a medical emergency and requires immediate intervention to prevent bowel infarction.

Intestinal Lymphangiectasia

Definition: A disorder characterized by dilated lymphatic vessels in the intestinal wall, leading to protein loss.

Pathophysiology: Abnormal development or obstruction of lymphatic vessels.

Signs and Symptoms: Protein-losing enteropathy, diarrhea, malabsorption, edema.

Causes/Risk Factors: Primary (congenital) or secondary (due to conditions like Crohn's disease).

Medical Management: Dietary modifications, nutritional supplements, and medications to reduce inflammation.

Surgical Management: Not typically indicated; focused on managing underlying causes.

Prognosis: Variable; depends on the extent of lymphatic involvement and underlying conditions.

Interesting Fact: Intestinal lymphangiectasia is a rare disorder and often requires a multidisciplinary approach for management.

Intestinal Obstruction in Neonates

Definition: Intestinal obstruction in neonates refers to a blockage in the digestive tract that prevents the normal flow of food, fluid, or gas.

Pathophysiology: Various congenital abnormalities, such as malrotation, atresia, or meconium ileus, can cause intestinal obstruction in neonates.

Signs and Symptoms: Abdominal distension, vomiting, failure to pass stool, feeding difficulties, and signs of dehydration.

Causes/Risk Factors: Congenital anomalies, genetic factors, or maternal factors during pregnancy might contribute to the development of intestinal obstructions in neonates.

Medical Management: Nasogastric decompression, intravenous fluids, and antibiotics. Surgical intervention is often necessary to correct the underlying anatomical defect.

Surgical Management: Surgery to remove or repair the obstructed portion of the intestine and restore normal bowel continuity.

Prognosis: Prognosis depends on the underlying cause and how quickly the condition is diagnosed and treated. Prompt surgical intervention often leads to a good outcome.

Interesting Fact: Intestinal obstructions in neonates are relatively common and require immediate medical attention to prevent complications.

Intrabdominal Abscess

Definition: An intrabdominal abscess is a localized collection of pus within the abdominal cavity, often resulting from untreated infections.

Pathophysiology: Infections, such as appendicitis or diverticulitis, can progress to abscess formation due to bacterial proliferation.

Signs and Symptoms: Fever, localized abdominal pain, swelling, tenderness, and signs of sepsis.

Causes/Risk Factors: Previous abdominal surgeries, inflammatory bowel disease, and immunosuppression increase the risk.

Medical Management: Intravenous antibiotics, drainage of the abscess guided by imaging, and supportive care.

Surgical Management: Drainage of the abscess either through open surgery or laparoscopic procedures.

Prognosis: Prognosis is generally good with timely drainage and appropriate antibiotic therapy.

Interesting Fact: Intrabdominal abscesses can lead to serious complications if left untreated, such as peritonitis and septic shock.

Irritable Bowel Syndrome (IBS)

Definition: Functional gastrointestinal disorder characterized by abdominal pain and altered bowel habits.

Pathophysiology: Complex, involving abnormal gut motility, hypersensitivity, and psychosocial factors.

Signs and Symptoms: Abdominal pain, diarrhea, constipation, bloating, mucus in stool.

Causes/Risk Factors: Genetic predisposition, gut-brain axis dysregulation, food intolerances.

Medical Management: Dietary modifications, antispasmodic medications, psychological therapies.

Surgical Management: Not curable by surgery; reserved for complications or refractory cases.

Prognosis: Chronic, but symptoms can often be managed with lifestyle changes.

Interesting Fact: IBS is a common gastrointestinal disorder, affecting about 10-15% of the global population.

Ischemic Colitis

Definition: Inflammation of the colon due to inadequate blood supply, leading to tissue damage.

Pathophysiology: Reduced blood flow to the colon, often due to vascular diseases.

Signs and Symptoms: Abdominal pain, bloody diarrhea, fever, urgency.

Causes/Risk Factors: Atherosclerosis, vasculitis, thrombosis, hypoperfusion.

Medical Management: IV fluids, antibiotics, bowel rest.

Surgical Management: Colectomy in severe cases, especially if gangrene or perforation occurs.

Prognosis: Variable; depends on the extent of ischemia and underlying causes.

Interesting Fact: Ischemic colitis can mimic other gastrointestinal conditions and often requires careful evaluation for diagnosis.

Islet Cell Tumor (Pancreatic Neuroendocrine Tumor)

Definition: Tumor arising from the pancreatic islet cells, often secreting hormones.

Pathophysiology: Uncontrolled growth of hormone-producing cells in the pancreas.

Signs and Symptoms: Hormone-related symptoms (such as hypoglycemia, diarrhea, flushing), abdominal pain.

Causes/Risk Factors: Genetic mutations, multiple endocrine neoplasia type 1 (MEN1) syndrome.

Medical Management: Somatostatin analogs, targeted therapy, chemotherapy.

Surgical Management: Tumor resection, sometimes with removal of affected organs (like the pancreas or duodenum).

Prognosis: Variable, depending on the tumor size, hormone production, and extent of spread; generally better than pancreatic adenocarcinoma.

Interesting Fact: Islet cell tumors can produce various hormones, leading to a range of symptoms, and often require a multidisciplinary approach for management.

Kawasaki Disease

Definition: Kawasaki disease is an autoimmune condition primarily affecting children, causing inflammation in blood vessels throughout the body.

Pathophysiology: The exact cause is unknown; it is believed to involve an abnormal immune response triggered by infections.

Signs and Symptoms: High fever, rash, red eyes, swollen hands and feet, and swollen lymph nodes.

Causes/Risk Factors: Often follows a viral infection, but specific triggers are unclear.

Medical Management: Intravenous immunoglobulin (IVIG), aspirin, and supportive care to reduce inflammation.

Surgical Management: Rarely needed; may involve interventions for coronary artery aneurysms in severe cases.

Prognosis: Prognosis is generally good with prompt treatment. Cardiac complications are a concern in untreated or severe cases.

Interesting Fact: Kawasaki disease is the leading cause of acquired heart disease in children in developed countries.

Klippel-Trenaunay Syndrome

Definition: Klippel-Trenaunay syndrome is a rare congenital disorder characterized by vascular malformations, soft tissue hypertrophy, and bone overgrowth.

Pathophysiology: Abnormal development of blood vessels and tissues during fetal growth.

Signs and Symptoms: Port-wine stains on the skin, varicose veins, limb overgrowth, and lymphatic malformations.

Causes/Risk Factors: Genetic mutations during embryonic development.

Medical Management: Symptomatic treatment, compression therapy, and laser therapy for skin lesions.

Surgical Management: Surgical interventions to manage complications like varicose veins or limb length discrepancies.

Prognosis: Prognosis varies based on the extent of complications. Management aims to improve quality of life.

Interesting Fact: Klippel-Trenaunay syndrome is a rare condition, and its exact cause remains unknown. Treatment is usually tailored to individual symptoms.

Langerhans Cell Histiocytosis

Definition: Rare disorder involving clonal proliferation of Langerhans cells, leading to tissue damage.

Pathophysiology: Abnormal proliferation of Langerhans cells, a type of immune cell.

Signs and Symptoms: Bone pain, skin rash, organ dysfunction based on involvement.

Causes/Risk Factors: Unknown; often sporadic.

Medical Management: Chemotherapy, immunotherapy, targeted therapy.

Surgical Management: Lesion excision in localized cases.

Prognosis: Variable; depends on the extent of disease and organ involvement.

Interesting Fact: Langerhans cell histiocytosis can affect people of all ages, but it is most common in children.

Leriche Syndrome

Definition: Leriche syndrome is a type of aortoiliac occlusive disease characterized by atherosclerosis leading to the obstruction of the distal aorta and both iliac arteries.

Pathophysiology: Atherosclerotic plaques in the aorta and iliac arteries cause reduced blood flow to the lower extremities.

Signs and Symptoms: Claudication, impotence, absent femoral pulses, and cold, pale legs.

Causes/Risk Factors: Atherosclerosis, smoking, hypertension, and diabetes.

Medical Management: Lifestyle modifications, antiplatelet medications, and supervised exercise programs.

Surgical Management: Aortoiliac bypass surgery or angioplasty and stenting.

Prognosis: Prognosis varies based on disease severity. Early intervention can improve symptoms and prevent complications.

Interesting Fact: Leriche syndrome is often called "aortoiliac occlusive disease of the elderly" and is more common in men.

Lipomas

Definition: Benign soft tissue tumors composed of fat cells.

Pathophysiology: Overgrowth of fat cells, forming a lump under the skin.

Signs and Symptoms: Soft, movable lump under the skin, often painless.

Causes/Risk Factors: Genetic predisposition, obesity.

Medical Management: Observation; surgical removal for cosmetic reasons or if symptomatic.

Surgical Management: Excision of the lipoma.

Prognosis: Excellent; benign and rarely recur after complete removal.

Interesting Fact: Lipomas are the most common soft tissue tumors, and they are usually harmless but can be removed if causing discomfort or for cosmetic reasons.

Liver Abscess

Definition: Collection of pus in the liver, often due to bacterial infection.

Pathophysiology: Bacterial infection in the liver tissue, leading to abscess formation.

Signs and Symptoms: Right upper quadrant pain, fever, jaundice, weight loss.

Causes/Risk Factors: Biliary tract infection, abdominal trauma, immunosuppression.

Medical Management: Antibiotics, drainage of the abscess if necessary.

Surgical Management: Percutaneous drainage or open surgical drainage for large or complicated abscesses.

Prognosis: Good with prompt medical intervention; can be life-threatening if untreated.

Interesting Fact: Liver abscesses can be single or multiple and are often caused by bacterial spread from other parts of the body.

Lung Abscess

Definition: A lung abscess is a localized collection of pus within the lung tissue, often resulting from bacterial infection.

Pathophysiology: Infection, aspiration, or pneumonia can lead to necrosis and cavitation in lung tissue, forming an abscess.

Signs and Symptoms: Cough with foul-smelling or bloody sputum, chest pain, fever, night sweats, and weight loss.

Causes/Risk Factors: Aspiration, pneumonia, immunosuppression, alcoholism, or lung obstruction.

Medical Management: Antibiotics targeting the causative bacteria, bronchoscopy for drainage, and supportive care.

Surgical Management: Surgical drainage or resection in severe or complicated cases.

Prognosis: Prognosis is generally good with prompt and appropriate antibiotic therapy. Delayed treatment can lead to complications.

Interesting Fact: Lung abscesses are often associated with aspiration of oral contents, especially in individuals with impaired consciousness.

Lung Cancer

Definition: Malignant tumor in the lungs.

Pathophysiology: Genetic mutations due to exposure to carcinogens, primarily smoking.

Signs and Symptoms: Persistent cough, hemoptysis, chest pain, weight loss, shortness of breath.

Causes/Risk Factors: Smoking, exposure to asbestos, radon, family history.

Medical Management: Chemotherapy, radiation therapy, targeted therapy, immunotherapy.

Surgical Management: Lobectomy (removal of a lobe), pneumonectomy (removal of an entire lung) in localized cases.

Prognosis: Varies widely based on the stage; early detection significantly improves outcomes.

Interesting Fact: Lung cancer is the leading cause of cancer-related deaths worldwide and is strongly associated with smoking.

Lymphedema

Definition: Swelling in one or more limbs, often due to the accumulation of lymphatic fluid.

Pathophysiology: Impaired lymphatic drainage, leading to fluid retention and swelling.

Signs and Symptoms: Swelling, heaviness, restricted range of motion, recurrent infections.

Causes/Risk Factors: Lymph node removal (often due to cancer treatment), lymphatic malformations.

Medical Management: Compression garments, manual lymphatic drainage, exercise.

Surgical Management: Lymphaticovenous anastomosis, lymph node transfer.

Prognosis: Chronic condition requiring lifelong management; can be managed effectively with appropriate measures.

Interesting Fact: Lymphedema is a common complication of cancer treatments like surgery and radiation therapy and requires ongoing care to prevent complications.

Lymphoepithelial Cyst

Definition: Benign cystic lesion often found in the parotid or submandibular salivary glands.

Pathophysiology: Cyst formation due to ductal obstruction and accumulation of saliva.

Signs and Symptoms: Palpable lump, usually asymptomatic; may cause discomfort if large.

Causes/Risk Factors: Ductal obstruction, salivary gland inflammation.

Medical Management: None; surgical excision if symptomatic.

Surgical Management: Complete excision of the cyst.

Prognosis: Excellent; recurrence is rare after complete removal.

Interesting Fact: Lymphoepithelial cysts are benign and do not have a risk of malignant transformation.

Malignant Melanoma

Definition: Aggressive skin cancer originating from melanocytes, often metastasizing to other organs.

Pathophysiology: Uncontrolled growth of melanocytes due to genetic mutations.

Signs and Symptoms: Irregular moles, changes in mole size, color, or shape, itching, bleeding.

Causes/Risk Factors: UV radiation exposure, genetic factors.

Medical Management: Excision, immunotherapy, targeted therapy.

Surgical Management: Wide local excision, lymph node biopsy, or dissection in advanced cases.

Prognosis: Variable; depends on the stage of melanoma and metastasis.

Interesting Fact: Malignant melanoma is one of the most aggressive forms of skin cancer and requires early detection and comprehensive treatment.

Mastitis

Definition: Inflammation of the breast tissue, often due to infection, occurring primarily in breastfeeding women.

Pathophysiology: Bacterial infection in the breast tissue, often entering through cracked nipples.

Signs and Symptoms: Breast pain, redness, swelling, flu-like symptoms.

Causes/Risk Factors: Bacterial infection (commonly Staphylococcus aureus), breastfeeding, cracked nipples.

Medical Management: Antibiotics, pain relief, warm compresses, continued breastfeeding.

Surgical Management: Drainage of abscess if present.

Prognosis: Good with appropriate medical management; can recur with subsequent infections.

Interesting Fact: Mastitis is a common condition in breastfeeding women and requires prompt treatment to prevent complications like abscess formation.

May-Thurner Syndrome

Definition: May-Thurner syndrome, also known as iliac vein compression syndrome, is a condition where the left common iliac vein is compressed by the right iliac artery, leading to deep vein thrombosis (DVT).

Pathophysiology: Compression of the left iliac vein causes reduced blood flow, increasing the risk of DVT.

Signs and Symptoms: Leg swelling, pain, and discoloration; symptoms similar to DVT.

Causes/Risk Factors: Anatomic variation, often seen in females.

Medical Management: Anticoagulant therapy for DVT, compression stockings, and lifestyle modifications.

Surgical Management: Venoplasty and stent placement to relieve iliac vein compression.

Prognosis: The prognosis is good with appropriate management, although there is a risk of DVT recurrence.

Interesting Fact: May-Thurner syndrome is more common in females and often presents in young to middle-aged adults.

Meckel's Diverticulum

Definition: Congenital pouch in the small intestine, a remnant of the omphalomesenteric duct.

Pathophysiology: Persistence of a fetal structure, leading to a blind pouch in the intestine.

Signs and Symptoms: Often asymptomatic; can cause abdominal pain, bleeding, or obstruction.

Causes/Risk Factors: Congenital anomaly, genetic factors.

Medical Management: Observation, symptomatic treatment for mild cases.

Surgical Management: Diverticulectomy (surgical removal of the diverticulum) for symptomatic or complicated cases.

Prognosis: Excellent after surgical removal; often asymptomatic and discovered incidentally.

Interesting Fact: Meckel's diverticulum is a common congenital anomaly, occurring in about 2% of the population.

Mediastinal Tumors

Definition: Mediastinal tumors are abnormal growths that develop in the mediastinum, the area in the middle of the chest containing the heart, large blood vessels, trachea, and esophagus.

Pathophysiology: Tumors can arise from various tissues in the mediastinum, including the thymus, lymph nodes, or neural tissues, leading to compression of nearby structures.

Signs and Symptoms: Chest pain, cough, difficulty swallowing, shortness of breath, and in some cases, symptoms related to hormonal imbalances if the tumor affects endocrine tissues.

Causes/Risk Factors: Unknown; some tumors are associated with specific conditions, while others occur sporadically.

Medical Management: Depending on the type of tumor, treatment may include surgery, chemotherapy, radiation therapy, or targeted therapies.

Surgical Management: Complete or partial removal of the tumor, often requiring complex surgical techniques due to proximity to vital structures.

Prognosis: Prognosis varies widely based on the type of tumor, its location, and the extent of surgical resection. Early diagnosis and comprehensive treatment improve outcomes.

Interesting Fact: Mediastinal tumors can be challenging to diagnose due to their location and diverse origins, necessitating a multidisciplinary approach for accurate evaluation and management.

Mediastinitis

Definition: Mediastinitis is inflammation of the tissues in the mediastinum, often due to infection.

Pathophysiology: Infections, trauma, or surgery can lead to the spread of bacteria to the mediastinal space.

Signs and Symptoms: Chest pain, fever, difficulty swallowing, and rapid heart rate.

Causes/Risk Factors: Post-surgical complications, esophageal perforation, or deep neck infections.

Medical Management: Intravenous antibiotics, drainage of infected fluid, and supportive care.

Surgical Management: Surgical drainage and debridement of infected tissues.

Prognosis: Prognosis depends on the underlying cause and timely intervention. Delayed treatment can lead to severe complications.

Interesting Fact: Mediastinitis can result from dental procedures, highlighting the interconnectedness of oral health and systemic well-being.

Mesenteric Ischemia

Definition: Reduced blood flow to the intestines, leading to tissue damage and potential gangrene.

Pathophysiology: Occlusion or narrowing of mesenteric arteries, causing inadequate blood supply to the intestines.

Signs and Symptoms: Severe abdominal pain, tenderness, vomiting, bloody stools, signs of shock.

Causes/Risk Factors: Atherosclerosis, embolism, thrombosis, mesenteric venous thrombosis.

Medical Management: Intravenous fluids, anticoagulants, addressing underlying causes.

Surgical Management: Revascularization procedures, bowel resection for necrotic tissue.

Prognosis: Variable, depending on the extent of ischemia and timely intervention.

Interesting Fact: Mesenteric ischemia is a medical emergency and requires immediate intervention to prevent bowel infarction.

Mesothelioma

Definition: Malignant tumor originating from the mesothelial cells, often associated with asbestos exposure.

Pathophysiology: Uncontrolled cell growth in the mesothelial lining of organs, usually the lungs or abdomen.

Signs and Symptoms: Shortness of breath, chest pain, abdominal swelling, weight loss.

Causes/Risk Factors: Asbestos exposure, radiation exposure, genetic factors.

Medical Management: Chemotherapy, radiation therapy, targeted therapy.

Surgical Management: Surgical resection (if operable) or palliative procedures for symptom relief.

Prognosis: Poor; often diagnosed at an advanced stage with limited treatment options.

Interesting Fact: Mesothelioma has a long latency period, often appearing several decades after asbestos exposure.

Mycotic Aneurysm

Definition: Mycotic aneurysm is a localized dilation of an artery due to a bacterial or fungal infection.

Pathophysiology: Infection weakens the arterial wall, leading to aneurysm formation.

Signs and Symptoms: Fever, localized pain, pulsating mass, and signs of sepsis in severe cases.

Causes/Risk Factors: Bacterial endocarditis, intravenous drug use, or trauma leading to infection.

Medical Management: Intravenous antibiotics, control of sepsis, and monitoring for signs of rupture.

Surgical Management: Aneurysm repair, often involving graft placement, after controlling the infection.

Prognosis: Prognosis depends on the underlying infection and timely intervention. Mortality rates can be high in severe cases.

Interesting Fact: Mycotic aneurysms are rare but can be life-threatening, requiring immediate medical and surgical attention.

Nasopharyngeal Carcinoma

Definition: Malignant tumor arising from the nasopharynx, often associated with Epstein-Barr virus (EBV) infection.

Pathophysiology: Uncontrolled cell growth in the nasopharyngeal tissue.

Signs and Symptoms: Nasal congestion, epistaxis, hearing loss, lymphadenopathy.

Causes/Risk Factors: Epstein-Barr virus infection, genetic factors, environmental factors.

Medical Management: Chemotherapy, radiation therapy.

Surgical Management: Surgical resection in select cases; often combined with other treatments.

Prognosis: Variable; depends on the stage and extent of the tumor.

Interesting Fact: Nasopharyngeal carcinoma is rare in most parts of the world but relatively common in certain regions, particularly in Southeast Asia.

Necrotizing Enterocolitis (NEC)

Definition: Inflammatory bowel disease primarily affecting premature infants, leading to tissue death in the intestines.

Pathophysiology: Impaired blood flow to the intestines, bacterial invasion, and inflammation.

Signs and Symptoms: Abdominal distension, bloody stools, lethargy, feeding intolerance in premature infants.

Causes/Risk Factors: Prematurity, low birth weight, formula feeding in preterm infants.

Medical Management: NPO (nothing by mouth), intravenous nutrition, antibiotics, close monitoring.

Surgical Management: Resection of necrotic intestine, temporary ostomy in severe cases.

Prognosis: Variable, depending on the extent of necrosis and timely intervention.

Interesting Fact: NEC is a leading cause of morbidity and mortality in premature infants and requires prompt medical and surgical evaluation.

Necrotizing Fasciitis

Definition: Severe soft tissue infection characterized by rapid spreading of necrosis in the fascial plane.

Pathophysiology: Bacterial infection leading to tissue destruction and necrosis.

Signs and Symptoms: Severe pain, swelling, redness, fever, crepitus (gas under the skin).

Causes/Risk Factors: Bacterial infection (commonly group A Streptococcus), immunosuppression, trauma.

Medical Management: Broad-spectrum antibiotics, supportive care.

Surgical Management: Surgical debridement, sometimes multiple surgeries, amputation in severe cases.

Prognosis: Poor if not treated promptly; high mortality rate.

Interesting Fact: Necrotizing fasciitis is a rapidly progressing infection that can spread within hours, leading to extensive tissue damage.

Necrotizing Soft Tissue Infections

Definition: Necrotizing soft tissue infections are severe bacterial infections that cause rapid destruction of skin, muscles, and underlying tissues.

Pathophysiology: Bacteria, often group A Streptococcus or Staphylococcus aureus, invade and release toxins, leading to tissue necrosis and systemic toxicity.

Signs and Symptoms: Severe pain, swelling, redness, fever, and rapidly spreading areas of skin discoloration.

Causes/Risk Factors: Breaks in the skin (cuts, burns, insect bites) allow bacteria to enter, and immunocompromised individuals are at higher risk.

Medical Management: Intravenous antibiotics, aggressive wound care, and often surgical debridement of necrotic tissue.

Surgical Management: Surgical exploration and debridement to remove necrotic tissue and control the infection's spread.

Prognosis: Mortality rates are high if not promptly treated. Early recognition and intervention are crucial.

Interesting Fact: Necrotizing soft tissue infections are sometimes referred to as "flesh-eating bacteria," highlighting their rapid tissue destruction.

Neuroblastoma

Definition: Malignant tumor arising from neural crest cells, often found in adrenal glands or along the spine.

Pathophysiology: Abnormal growth of immature nerve cells.

Signs and Symptoms: Abdominal mass, pain, changes in bowel habits, weakness.

Causes/Risk Factors: Genetic mutations, often sporadic.

Medical Management: Chemotherapy, surgery, radiation therapy.

Surgical Management: Tumor resection; may require extensive surgery in advanced cases.

Prognosis: Variable, depending on the stage and age of the patient; good outcomes with early detection in children.

Interesting Fact: Neuroblastoma is a common childhood cancer, usually diagnosed in infants and young children, and often requires a multimodal approach to treatment.

Neuroendocrine Tumors

Definition: Neuroendocrine tumors (NETs) are a group of rare tumors that arise from cells of the neuroendocrine system.

Pathophysiology: NETs develop from neuroendocrine cells that release hormones. They can occur in various organs, including the gastrointestinal tract and lungs.

Signs and Symptoms: Symptoms depend on the location and hormone production but may include flushing, diarrhea, abdominal pain, wheezing, and weight loss.

Causes/Risk Factors: Genetic mutations, certain endocrine disorders, and exposure to certain chemicals might increase the risk.

Medical Management: Somatostatin analogs, chemotherapy, targeted therapy, and in some cases, peptide receptor radionuclide therapy (PRRT).

Surgical Management: Surgical removal of localized tumors. In metastatic cases, surgery might be combined with other treatments.

Prognosis: Prognosis varies widely based on the tumor location, size, and stage at diagnosis. Some NETs are slow-growing and manageable, while others can be aggressive.

Interesting Fact: NETs are often called "carcinoid tumors," but this term is now being replaced by the more encompassing term "neuroendocrine tumors."

Ovarian Cyst

Definition: Fluid-filled sacs in or on the ovaries, often benign but can cause symptoms or complications.

Pathophysiology: Follicles or eggs in the ovaries fail to rupture or release the egg, leading to cyst formation.

Signs and Symptoms: Pelvic pain, bloating, changes in menstrual cycle, pain during intercourse.

Causes/Risk Factors: Hormonal imbalances, endometriosis, polycystic ovary syndrome (PCOS).

Medical Management: Observation, hormonal contraceptives, pain management.

Surgical Management: Cystectomy (surgical removal of the cyst), oophorectomy in severe or recurrent cases.

Prognosis: Generally good; most cysts are benign and resolve on their own.

Interesting Fact: Ovarian cysts are common and often asymptomatic, but can cause pain or complications if they grow large or rupture.

Paget-Schroetter Syndrome (Effort Thrombosis)

Definition: Paget-Schroetter syndrome is a type of deep vein thrombosis (DVT) occurring in the upper extremity, often due to repetitive arm motion.

Pathophysiology: Compression of the subclavian vein by the clavicle and first rib causes blood clot formation.

Signs and Symptoms: Swelling, pain, and discoloration in the affected arm; can be associated with a history of strenuous arm activity.

Causes/Risk Factors: Repetitive arm motion, anatomical abnormalities, or thoracic outlet syndrome.

Medical Management: Anticoagulant therapy, compression therapy, and lifestyle modifications.

Surgical Management: Thrombolysis, venoplasty, or first rib resection in severe cases.

Prognosis: The prognosis is good with early diagnosis and appropriate management.

Interesting Fact: Paget-Schroetter syndrome is often seen in athletes or individuals with repetitive overhead arm movements.

Pancreatic Cancer

Definition: Malignant tumor in the pancreas.

Pathophysiology: Genetic mutations, often asymptomatic until advanced stages.

Signs and Symptoms: Abdominal pain, jaundice, weight loss, digestive problems.

Causes/Risk Factors: Smoking, family history, diabetes, certain genetic syndromes.

Medical Management: Chemotherapy, radiation therapy, immunotherapy.

Surgical Management: Whipple procedure (pancreaticoduodenectomy) or distal pancreatectomy in localized cases.

Prognosis: Poor prognosis due to late-stage diagnosis in many cases.

Interesting Fact: Pancreatic cancer is often diagnosed at an advanced stage, leading to a high mortality rate.

Pancreatic Pseudocyst

Definition: Collection of fluid, enzymes, and tissue debris in or around the pancreas, forming a pseudocyst.

Pathophysiology: Leakage of pancreatic enzymes and fluid due to pancreatitis or pancreatic trauma.

Signs and Symptoms: Abdominal pain, fullness, nausea, vomiting, palpable abdominal mass.

Causes/Risk Factors: Pancreatitis, pancreatic trauma, complications of pancreatic surgery.

Medical Management: Observation for asymptomatic small pseudocysts, drainage for symptomatic or large pseudocysts.

Surgical Management: Percutaneous drainage, endoscopic drainage, cystgastrostomy, or cystjejunostomy in refractory cases.

Prognosis: Variable, depending on the size and location of the pseudocyst; can resolve spontaneously or require intervention.

Interesting Fact: Pancreatic pseudocysts can develop as a complication of acute or chronic pancreatitis and may require intervention if they cause symptoms or complications.

Pancreatitis

Definition: Inflammation of the pancreas.

Pathophysiology: Autodigestion of the pancreas by its own enzymes, leading to inflammation and tissue damage.

Signs and Symptoms: Severe abdominal pain, nausea, vomiting, fever, jaundice.

Causes/Risk Factors: Alcohol abuse, gallstones, high triglycerides, certain medications.

Medical Management: Fasting, IV fluids, pain control. Management of underlying causes.

Surgical Management: Rarely required, may be considered in severe cases with complications like necrosis.

Prognosis: Variable, depending on the cause and severity.

Interesting Fact: Pancreatitis can be acute (sudden onset) or chronic (persistent inflammation), both of which can be serious and require medical attention.

Parathyroid Adenoma

Definition: Benign tumor in the parathyroid gland, leading to excessive production of parathyroid hormone (PTH).

Pathophysiology: Abnormal growth of parathyroid cells causing increased PTH secretion.

Signs and Symptoms: Hypercalcemia, kidney stones, bone pain, fatigue.

Causes/Risk Factors: Unknown; often sporadic.

Medical Management: Monitoring calcium levels, and medications to control calcium levels.

Surgical Management: Parathyroidectomy (removal of the affected parathyroid gland).

Prognosis: Excellent with surgery; recurrence is rare after complete removal.

Interesting Fact: Parathyroid adenomas are a common cause of primary hyperparathyroidism, leading to calcium imbalances in the body.

Parathyroid Cancer

Definition: Malignant tumor originating from the parathyroid glands, leading to excessive production of parathyroid hormone (PTH).

Pathophysiology: Uncontrolled cell growth in the parathyroid tissue.

Signs and Symptoms: Hypercalcemia, kidney stones, bone pain, fatigue.

Causes/Risk Factors: Genetic mutations, radiation exposure.

Medical Management: Monitoring calcium levels, and medications to control calcium levels.

Surgical Management: Parathyroidectomy with possible neck dissection.

Prognosis: Guarded; often diagnosed at an advanced stage due to limited symptoms.

Interesting Fact: Parathyroid cancer is rare, comprising less than 1% of all cases of primary hyperparathyroidism.

Parathyroid Disorders

Definition: Disorders affecting the parathyroid glands, leading to abnormal calcium levels.

Pathophysiology: Hyperparathyroidism (excessive PTH secretion) or hypoparathyroidism (insufficient PTH secretion).

Signs and Symptoms: Hypercalcemia, kidney stones, bone pain (hyperparathyroidism), muscle cramps, seizures (hypoparathyroidism).

Causes/Risk Factors: Tumors, genetic factors, surgery.

Medical Management: Surgery for tumors, medications to regulate calcium levels.

Surgical Management: Parathyroidectomy (removal of abnormal parathyroid glands).

Prognosis: Generally good with appropriate management.

Interesting Fact: There are usually four parathyroid glands, located behind the thyroid gland, regulating calcium metabolism in the body.

Parathyroid Hyperplasia

Definition: Parathyroid hyperplasia is a condition in which all four parathyroid glands become enlarged and overactive.

Pathophysiology: Uncontrolled growth of cells in the parathyroid glands, leading to excessive production of parathyroid hormone.

Signs and Symptoms: High calcium levels, fatigue, weakness, and bone pain.

Causes/Risk Factors: Genetic predisposition, certain genetic syndromes, and radiation exposure.

Medical Management: Managing hypercalcemia, medications, and close monitoring of calcium levels.

Surgical Management: Parathyroidectomy to remove enlarged glands.

Prognosis: The prognosis is excellent after successful surgery. Calcium levels normalize after the affected glands are removed.

Interesting Fact: Parathyroid hyperplasia is a common cause of primary hyperparathyroidism, a condition characterized by excessive parathyroid hormone production.

Partial Splenectomy

Definition: Partial splenectomy involves removing a portion of the spleen while preserving the remaining healthy tissue. It is performed to treat conditions where only a specific area of the spleen is affected.

Pathophysiology: Partial splenectomy is indicated when there's localized damage or disease within the spleen, allowing the preservation of functional splenic tissue.

Signs and Symptoms: Varied, depending on the underlying condition. Symptoms may include pain, tenderness, or signs of anemia or infections if the affected spleen area impacts blood filtration or immune function.

Causes/Risk Factors: Trauma, focal infections, cysts, or tumors that affect specific areas of the spleen, leaving the rest of the organ functional.

Medical Management: Evaluation through imaging studies and blood tests to assess the extent of the spleen's involvement and the potential for partial splenectomy.

Surgical Management: During the procedure, the surgeon carefully removes the affected portion of the spleen, leaving healthy tissue intact. Preserving functional spleen tissue is essential to maintain immune functions.

Prognosis: Preservation of partial splenic function often leads to improved overall health and reduced symptoms related to the underlying condition.

Interesting Fact: Partial splenectomy strikes a balance between addressing the specific issue within the spleen and preserving enough functional tissue to maintain essential immune functions.

Pectus Excavatum

Definition: Pectus excavatum, also known as funnel chest, is a congenital deformity where the breastbone sinks into the chest, creating a sunken appearance.

Pathophysiology: Abnormal growth of the costal cartilages and ribs leads to the depression of the sternum.

Signs and Symptoms: Sunken chest, shortness of breath, chest pain, and heart palpitations.

Causes/Risk Factors: Genetic factors; often appear during adolescence during the growth spurt.

Medical Management: Observation in mild cases, chest wall exercises, and in severe cases, the use of chest braces during growth.

Surgical Management: Nuss procedure (minimally invasive surgery involving placement of a curved metal bar under the sternum) or Ravitch procedure (open surgery to correct the chest deformity).

Prognosis: Prognosis is excellent after surgical correction. Early intervention can prevent potential cardiac and respiratory issues.

Interesting Fact: Pectus excavatum can affect self-esteem due to the visible deformity, especially during adolescence. Surgical correction can significantly improve body image and confidence.

Pelvic Organ Prolapse

Definition: Descend or bulging of one or more pelvic organs (uterus, bladder, rectum) into the vaginal canal.

Pathophysiology: Weakness or damage to pelvic support tissues.

Signs and Symptoms: Vaginal bulge, discomfort, urinary or fecal incontinence.

Causes/Risk Factors: Childbirth, aging, obesity, connective tissue disorders.

Medical Management: Pelvic floor physical therapy, pessaries (vaginal devices).

Surgical Management: Pelvic organ suspension, mesh repair.

Prognosis: Variable; depends on the extent of prolapse and overall health.

Interesting Fact: Pelvic organ prolapse is a common condition affecting women, especially after childbirth and during menopause.

Peptic Ulcers

Definition: Erosion of the stomach or duodenal lining.

Pathophysiology: Imbalance between stomach acid and protective mucus in the stomach lining.

Signs and Symptoms: Burning epigastric pain, bloating, nausea, vomiting, weight loss.

Causes/Risk Factors: Helicobacter pylori infection, NSAID use, stress.

Medical Management: Antacids, proton pump inhibitors, antibiotics for H. pylori eradication.

Surgical Management: Rarely required; reserved for complications like perforation or obstruction.

Prognosis: Good with treatment but can recur if underlying causes are not addressed.

Interesting Fact: Most peptic ulcers are caused by H. pylori bacteria and can be effectively treated with antibiotics.

Perianal Abscess

Definition: Collection of pus near the anus.

Pathophysiology: Infection of anal glands or hair follicles.

Signs and Symptoms: Pain, swelling, redness, discharge.

Causes/Risk Factors: Bacterial infection.

Medical Management: Incision and drainage, antibiotics.

Surgical Management: Drainage of the abscess.

Prognosis: Generally good with proper drainage and antibiotics.

Interesting Fact: Perianal abscesses are common and can recur if not completely drained.

Peripheral Artery Disease (PAD)

Definition: Narrowing or blockage of arteries outside the heart, usually in the legs.

Pathophysiology: Atherosclerosis, plaque buildup in the arteries, leading to reduced blood flow.

Signs and Symptoms: Claudication (leg pain while walking), leg weakness, poor wound healing.

Causes/Risk Factors: Smoking, diabetes, hypertension, high cholesterol.

Medical Management: Lifestyle modifications, antiplatelet medications, statins.

Surgical Management: Angioplasty with stent placement, bypass surgery in severe cases.

Prognosis: Depends on the severity and extent of arterial blockages.

Interesting Fact: PAD is a significant risk factor for heart attack and stroke.

Peritonitis

Definition: Inflammation of the peritoneum, the lining of the abdominal cavity.

Pathophysiology: Bacterial infection, often due to perforation of the gastrointestinal tract.

Signs and Symptoms: Severe abdominal pain, tenderness, fever, vomiting.

Causes/Risk Factors: Gastrointestinal perforation, appendicitis, diverticulitis.

Medical Management: Intravenous antibiotics, supportive care, addressing underlying causes.

Surgical Management: Surgical repair of the perforation, and drainage of infected fluid.

Prognosis: Variable, depends on the extent of infection and timely intervention.

Interesting Fact: Peritonitis is a medical emergency and requires immediate surgical evaluation and intervention to prevent systemic complications.

Pilonidal Cyst

Definition: Cyst or abscess near the cleft of the buttocks, often containing hair and skin debris.

Pathophysiology: Hair penetration into the skin, leading to inflammation and abscess formation.

Signs and Symptoms: Pain, swelling, redness, drainage of pus.

Causes/Risk Factors: Friction or prolonged sitting, obesity, excessive body hair.

Medical Management: Incision and drainage, antibiotics, hygiene measures.

Surgical Management: Excision of the cyst and sinus tracts, wound closure.

Prognosis: Good with appropriate management; recurrence can occur without proper care.

Interesting Fact: Pilonidal cysts are more common in young adults and can be recurrent if not effectively treated.

Pilonidal Disease

Definition: Cyst or abscess near the tailbone (coccyx) that often contains hair and skin debris.

Pathophysiology: Hair penetration into the skin triggers an inflammatory response, forming a cyst or abscess.

Signs and Symptoms: Pain, swelling, redness, drainage of pus or blood.

Causes/Risk Factors: Ingrown hair, prolonged sitting, obesity, excessive body hair.

Medical Management: Incision and drainage, antibiotics. Recurrent cases may require surgery.

Surgical Management: Surgical excision of the cyst or sinus tract.

Prognosis: Generally good with appropriate management.

Interesting Fact: Pilonidal disease is often referred to as "jeep driver's disease" due to its historical association with military personnel who spent long hours driving in rough terrain.

Pleural Effusion

Definition: Accumulation of fluid in the pleural cavity (space between the lungs and chest wall).

Pathophysiology: Imbalance in fluid production and absorption in the pleural space.

Signs and Symptoms: Shortness of breath, chest pain, cough, decreased breath sounds.

Causes/Risk Factors: Infections, heart failure, malignancy, liver or kidney disease.

Medical Management: Thoracentesis (fluid drainage), underlying cause treatment.

Surgical Management: Pleurodesis (inducing pleural inflammation to prevent fluid accumulation), thoracic surgery in recurrent or complicated cases.

Prognosis: Depends on the underlying cause; good with timely and appropriate intervention.

Interesting Fact: Pleural effusion can be a complication of various medical conditions and often requires careful evaluation to determine the cause.

Pleuroparenchymal Fibroelastosis (PPFE)

Definition: PPFE is a rare interstitial lung disease characterized by fibrosis of pleural and subpleural lung tissues.

Pathophysiology: Abnormal wound healing processes lead to fibrosis, thickening the pleural and subpleural regions of the lungs.

Signs and Symptoms: Progressive shortness of breath, dry cough, and reduced exercise tolerance.

Causes/Risk Factors: Unknown; often idiopathic.

Medical Management: Oxygen therapy, immunosuppressive drugs, and lung transplantation in severe cases.

Surgical Management: Lung transplantation.

Prognosis: Prognosis is variable. Lung transplantation can be curative in select cases.

Interesting Fact: PPFE predominantly affects the upper lobes of the lungs, leading to unique radiological patterns.

Pneumothorax

Definition: Pneumothorax is the presence of air in the pleural space, causing lung collapse.

Pathophysiology: This can occur spontaneously or due to trauma, leading to a change in the balance between intrapleural pressure and lung elasticity.

Signs and Symptoms: Sudden chest pain, shortness of breath, rapid breathing, and decreased breath sounds on the affected side.

Causes/Risk Factors: Trauma, underlying lung diseases (such as COPD), or spontaneous without an apparent cause (primary spontaneous pneumothorax).

Medical Management: Small pneumothoraces may resolve on their own; large or recurrent cases may require chest tube insertion to remove air.

Surgical Management: Thoracoscopic surgery (video-assisted thoracoscopic surgery, VATS) or open surgery to repair blebs, pleurectomy, or pleurodesis.

Prognosis: Prognosis is generally good, especially with prompt treatment. Recurrence risk exists, especially in individuals with underlying lung conditions.

Interesting Fact: Tall, thin individuals, especially smokers, are at higher risk for spontaneous pneumothorax due to the prevalence of blebs on their lungs.

Polycystic Liver Disease

Definition: Genetic disorder characterized by the growth of numerous cysts in the liver.

Pathophysiology: Abnormal development of bile ducts leading to cyst formation.

Signs and Symptoms: Abdominal pain, hepatomegaly, complications like infection or bleeding.

Causes/Risk Factors: Genetic mutations, often autosomal dominant.

Medical Management: Symptomatic relief, monitoring for complications.

Surgical Management: Cyst fenestration, and liver resection in severe cases.

Prognosis: Variable; depends on the extent of cystic involvement and associated complications.

Interesting Fact: Polycystic liver disease can occur as an isolated condition or be part of a syndrome involving multiple organs.

Popliteal Artery Aneurysm

Definition: Popliteal artery aneurysm is the dilation of the popliteal artery, usually behind the knee.

Pathophysiology: Weakness in the arterial wall leads to bulging and potential rupture.

Signs and Symptoms: Often asymptomatic; pulsating mass behind the knee, leg pain, or limb-threatening ischemia if ruptured.

Causes/Risk Factors: Atherosclerosis, genetic factors, and trauma.

Medical Management: Blood pressure control, surveillance for growth, and antiplatelet medications.

Surgical Management: Aneurysm repair through open surgery or endovascular techniques.

Prognosis: Prognosis after successful repair is generally good. Ruptured aneurysms have high mortality rates.

Interesting Fact: Popliteal artery aneurysms are the most common peripheral artery aneurysms, but they are still relatively rare.

Popliteal Artery Entrapment Syndrome

Definition: Popliteal artery entrapment syndrome is a condition where the popliteal artery is compressed by nearby muscles and tendons in the knee, restricting blood flow.

Pathophysiology: Abnormal positioning of muscles and arteries in the leg causes compression during physical activity.

Signs and Symptoms: Leg pain, cramping, and weakness during exercise; relieved by rest.

Causes/Risk Factors: Anatomical abnormalities, often seen in young athletes.

Medical Management: Physical therapy and exercise modification.

Surgical Management: Surgery to release the entrapped artery if conservative measures fail.

Prognosis: Prognosis is excellent with surgical intervention, allowing individuals to resume normal activities.

Interesting Fact: Popliteal artery entrapment syndrome is more common.

Portal Hypertension

Definition: Portal hypertension is an increase in blood pressure within the portal vein system, often due to liver cirrhosis.

Pathophysiology: Liver dysfunction causes resistance to blood flow in the portal veins, leading to increased pressure.

Signs and Symptoms: Enlarged spleen, ascites, varicose veins in the esophagus (esophageal varices), and abdominal discomfort.

Causes/Risk Factors: Liver cirrhosis, hepatitis, or other liver diseases.

Medical Management: Medications to reduce portal pressure, dietary changes, and management of underlying liver disease.

Surgical Management: Transjugular intrahepatic portosystemic shunt (TIPS) or liver transplantation in severe cases.

Prognosis: The prognosis depends on the underlying liver disease. Severe cases can lead to life-threatening complications.

Interesting Fact: Portal hypertension can lead to the development of portosystemic collaterals, which are abnormal blood vessels bypassing the liver.

Primary Spontaneous Pneumothorax

Definition: Primary spontaneous pneumothorax occurs without any underlying lung disease or trauma.

Pathophysiology: Rupture of small blebs (air-filled sacs) on the lung surface leads to air leakage into the pleural space.

Signs and Symptoms: Sudden sharp chest pain, shortness of breath, and decreased breath sounds on the affected side.

Causes/Risk Factors: Often idiopathic, but smoking and genetic factors play a role.

Medical Management: Observation, oxygen therapy, or chest tube insertion.

Surgical Management: Video-assisted thoracoscopic surgery (VATS) to remove blebs and create pleurodesis.

Prognosis: Prognosis is generally good, especially with timely intervention. Recurrence risk exists, especially in smokers.

Interesting Fact: Tall, thin individuals, particularly males, are at higher risk for primary spontaneous pneumothorax, emphasizing the role of body morphology.

Pseudomyxoma Peritonei

Definition: A rare condition characterized by the accumulation of mucinous fluid in the peritoneal cavity due to a ruptured tumor.

Pathophysiology: The rupture of a mucinous tumor (often appendiceal) leads to the spread of mucinous material in the abdominal cavity.

Signs and Symptoms: Abdominal distension, pain, hernias, bowel obstruction.

Causes/Risk Factors: Mucinous tumors of the appendix or other organs.

Medical Management: Chemotherapy, sometimes intraperitoneal chemotherapy.

Surgical Management: Cytoreductive surgery, peritonectomy, hyperthermic intraperitoneal chemotherapy (HIPEC).

Prognosis: Variable; long-term survival possible with aggressive surgical management.

Interesting Fact: Pseudomyxoma peritonei requires complex surgical procedures and a multidisciplinary approach for effective management.

Pulmonary Embolism

Definition: Pulmonary embolism (PE) is a sudden blockage in one of the pulmonary arteries in the lungs, usually caused by blood clots that travel to the lungs from the legs or other parts of the body (deep vein thrombosis).

Pathophysiology: Blood clots or fat emboli travel through the bloodstream and lodge in the pulmonary arteries, obstructing blood flow to the lungs.

Signs and Symptoms: Shortness of breath, chest pain (especially upon breathing or coughing), rapid heart rate, cough that may produce bloody or blood-streaked sputum.

Causes/Risk Factors: Deep vein thrombosis, surgery, prolonged immobility, cancer, obesity, smoking, and certain genetic conditions.

Medical Management: Anticoagulants (blood thinners), thrombolytic therapy, oxygen therapy, and sometimes embolectomy in severe cases.

Surgical Management: Embolectomy (surgical removal of the clot) in life-threatening situations or when medications are ineffective.

Prognosis: Prognosis depends on the size and location of the clot and how quickly it is diagnosed and treated. Prompt treatment significantly improves outcomes.

Interesting Fact: Pulmonary embolism is a medical emergency and can be fatal if not treated promptly, making early diagnosis crucial.

Pulmonary Fibrosis

Definition: Pulmonary fibrosis involves scarring of lung tissue, leading to decreased oxygen exchange.

Pathophysiology: Chronic inflammation or environmental exposures lead to lung tissue damage and fibrosis.

Signs and Symptoms: Shortness of breath, persistent cough, fatigue, and chest pain.

Causes/Risk Factors: Environmental factors (such as asbestos exposure), autoimmune diseases, and genetic predisposition.

Medical Management: Corticosteroids, immunosuppressive drugs, and oxygen therapy.

Surgical Management: Lung transplant in severe cases.

Prognosis: Prognosis varies. Lung transplant can significantly improve the quality of life.

Interesting Fact: Some cases of pulmonary fibrosis have been linked to specific medications and treatments, highlighting the importance of monitoring patients for potential side effects.

Pulmonary Sequestration

Definition: Pulmonary sequestration is a rare congenital malformation where a portion of lung tissue is isolated from the normal bronchial tree and blood supply.

Pathophysiology: Abnormal development during fetal growth leads to a non-functioning, isolated lung tissue mass.

Signs and Symptoms: Often asymptomatic; discovered incidentally during imaging. In some cases, recurrent respiratory infections or chest pain.

Causes/Risk Factors: Congenital anomaly; occurs during fetal development.

Medical Management: Observation in asymptomatic cases, surgical resection in symptomatic cases.

Surgical Management: Surgical removal of the sequestered lung tissue, usually performed with a thoracotomy or thoracoscopy.

Prognosis: Prognosis is excellent after surgical removal. Asymptomatic cases do not require intervention.

Interesting Fact: Pulmonary sequestration can receive its blood supply from systemic arteries, making it distinct from the surrounding normal lung tissue.

Pyloric Stenosis

Definition: Narrowing of the opening between the stomach and the small intestine (pylorus), leading to obstruction.

Pathophysiology: Hypertrophy and thickening of the pyloric muscles.

Signs and Symptoms: Non-bilious vomiting, visible peristalsis, failure to thrive.

Causes/Risk Factors: Unknown; often idiopathic.

Medical Management: Intravenous fluids, correction of electrolyte imbalances.

Surgical Management: Pyloromyotomy (surgical incision of the pyloric muscles).

Prognosis: Excellent with surgery; complications are rare.

Interesting Fact: Pyloric stenosis is a common cause of vomiting in infants and typically presents in the first few weeks of life.

Raynaud's Disease

Definition: Raynaud's disease is a condition where blood flow to certain parts of the body, usually fingers and toes, is reduced in response to cold or stress, leading to color changes and discomfort.

Pathophysiology: Blood vessel spasms, often triggered by cold or emotional stress, reduce blood flow temporarily.

Signs and Symptoms: Color changes in extremities (white, blue, and red), numbness, and tingling.

Causes/Risk Factors: The exact cause is unknown; can be primary (idiopathic) or secondary to other conditions.

Medical Management: Avoiding triggers, medications to dilate blood vessels, and managing underlying conditions in secondary cases.

Surgical Management: Sympathectomy in severe cases.

Prognosis: The prognosis is generally good, but severe cases can lead to complications like ulcers or tissue damage.

Interesting Fact: Raynaud's disease is more common in colder climates and affects more women than men. It often develops in young adults.

Rectal Cancer

Definition: Malignant tumor in the rectum, the final portion of the large intestine.

Pathophysiology: Uncontrolled cell growth in the rectal tissue, often starting as polyps.

Signs and Symptoms: Changes in bowel habits, blood in stool, abdominal pain, weight loss.

Causes/Risk Factors: Age, family history, inflammatory bowel disease, certain genetic syndromes.

Medical Management: Chemotherapy, radiation therapy, targeted therapy.

Surgical Management: Low anterior resection (surgical removal of the rectal tumor), colostomy in advanced cases.

Prognosis: Varies based on the stage and extent of spread; early detection improves outcomes.

Interesting Fact: Rectal cancer is often diagnosed through colonoscopies and requires a multidisciplinary approach for treatment.

Rectal Prolapse

Definition: Rectum protrudes through the anus.

Pathophysiology: Weakness in the rectal muscles and ligaments.

Signs and Symptoms: Visible protrusion, discomfort, mucus discharge, incontinence.

Causes/Risk Factors: Chronic constipation, childbirth, aging.

Medical Management: Dietary changes, pelvic floor exercises. Severe cases may require surgery.

Surgical Management: Rectopexy (surgery to secure the rectum) is the standard procedure.

Prognosis: Generally good with surgery, but recurrence is possible.

Interesting Fact: Rectal prolapse is more common in older adults and women who have had multiple childbirths.

Renal Artery Stenosis

Definition: Renal artery stenosis is the narrowing of one or both renal arteries, leading to reduced blood flow to the kidneys.

Pathophysiology: Atherosclerosis or fibromuscular dysplasia causes narrowing of the renal arteries.

Signs and Symptoms: Hypertension, decreased kidney function, and fluid retention.

Causes/Risk Factors: Atherosclerosis, fibromuscular dysplasia, or vasculitis.

Medical Management: Blood pressure medications, lifestyle modifications, and management of underlying conditions.

Surgical Management: Renal artery angioplasty and stent placement in select cases.

Prognosis: Prognosis depends on the cause and extent of stenosis. Timely intervention can prevent kidney damage.

Interesting Fact: Renal artery stenosis is a potentially reversible cause of hypertension, especially in younger individuals.

Renal Stones (Nephrolithiasis)

Definition: Formation of solid crystals in the kidneys, leading to stones.

Pathophysiology: Supersaturation of urine with mineral components like calcium, oxalate, or uric acid.

Signs and Symptoms: Flank pain, hematuria, urinary urgency.

Causes/Risk Factors: Dehydration, high dietary intake of certain minerals, genetic factors.

Medical Management: Hydration, pain management, medications to dissolve stones.

Surgical Management: Lithotripsy, ureteroscopy, or surgery for large or obstructive stones.

Prognosis: Generally good with treatment; recurrence is common without dietary modifications.

Interesting Fact: Certain dietary modifications, like reducing salt and animal protein intake, can help prevent kidney stones.

Retroperitoneal Fibrosis

Definition: Abnormal formation of fibrous tissue in the retroperitoneal space, often compressing nearby structures.

Pathophysiology: Idiopathic inflammation leading to fibrous tissue formation.

Signs and Symptoms: Flank pain, swelling, renal impairment, hypertension.

Causes/Risk Factors: Idiopathic, sometimes associated with certain medications or malignancies.

Medical Management: Corticosteroids, immunosuppressive drugs.

Surgical Management: Surgery to remove fibrous tissue and relieve compression.

Prognosis: Variable; relapses can occur.

Interesting Fact: Retroperitoneal fibrosis can be challenging to diagnose and may require a multidisciplinary approach for management.

Ruptured Abdominal Aortic Aneurysm (AAA)

Definition: AAA rupture occurs when a weakened and enlarged segment of the abdominal aorta tears, leading to massive internal bleeding.

Pathophysiology: Chronic high blood pressure, atherosclerosis, and genetic factors contribute to the weakening of the aortic wall.

Signs and Symptoms: Sudden, severe abdominal or back pain, hypotension, rapid pulse, and loss of consciousness.

Causes/Risk Factors: Hypertension, smoking, atherosclerosis, and family history of AAA.

Medical Management: Urgent volume resuscitation, blood transfusions, and controlling blood pressure.

Surgical Management: Emergency open surgical repair or endovascular stent grafting.

Prognosis: Mortality rates are high, but prompt surgical intervention improves the chances of survival.

Interesting Fact: AAAs are often asymptomatic until they rupture, making regular screening important for at-risk individuals.

Small Bowel Obstruction

Definition: Blockage of the small intestine, often due to adhesions or hernias.

Pathophysiology: Physical blockage of the intestine, preventing the passage of contents.

Signs and Symptoms: Abdominal pain, distension, vomiting, constipation.

Causes/Risk Factors: Adhesions, hernias, tumors, Crohn's disease.

Medical Management: NPO (nothing by mouth), IV fluids, nasogastric tube decompression.

Surgical Management: Surgery to remove the obstruction or repair hernias/adhesions.

Prognosis: Generally good with timely intervention, but complications can occur.

Interesting Fact: Adhesions, often from previous abdominal surgeries, are a common cause of small bowel obstruction.

Spigelian Hernia

Definition: Hernia that occurs along the linea semilunaris, often in the lower abdomen.

Pathophysiology: Weakness in the abdominal wall muscles, allowing protrusion of abdominal contents.

Signs and Symptoms: Bulge, discomfort, pain, especially during lifting or straining.

Causes/Risk Factors: Muscle weakness, obesity, previous surgery.

Medical Management: Supportive garments, lifestyle modifications.

Surgical Management: Hernia repair with mesh, sometimes laparoscopic surgery.

Prognosis: Good with surgical repair; can recur if underlying risk factors are not addressed.

Interesting Fact: Spigelian hernias are relatively rare and can be challenging to diagnose due to their location.

Spleen Biopsy

Definition: A spleen biopsy is a diagnostic procedure where a small sample of spleen tissue is removed and examined under a microscope to diagnose various conditions, including blood disorders and cancers.

Pathophysiology: The procedure helps identify abnormal cell growth, infections, or inflammatory conditions within the spleen tissue.

Signs and Symptoms: Spleen enlargement, unexplained weight loss, fever, night sweats, and general malaise, which might indicate underlying splenic abnormalities.

Causes/Risk Factors: Suspected blood disorders, infections, or malignancies where a definitive diagnosis is required.

Medical Management: Pre-biopsy evaluations, such as imaging studies and blood tests, to assess overall health and determine the need for the procedure.

Surgical Management: The biopsy can be performed through various techniques, including ultrasound-guided needle biopsy or open surgical biopsy, depending on the suspected condition and the location of the abnormality.

Prognosis: The prognosis depends on the underlying condition diagnosed through the biopsy. Early detection often leads to better outcomes.

Interesting Fact: Spleen biopsy is a valuable tool in diagnosing specific diseases, helping healthcare providers determine appropriate treatment plans for patients.

Splenectomy

Definition: Splenectomy is the surgical removal of the spleen, usually performed due to trauma, blood disorders, or splenic tumors.

Pathophysiology: Various conditions like splenic rupture, hematological disorders, or tumors can necessitate splenectomy. Removal of the spleen affects immune functions and blood filtration, leading to altered physiological processes.

Signs and Symptoms: Pain in the left upper abdomen, abdominal tenderness, signs of shock (in case of trauma), easy bruising, frequent infections, and anemia in certain blood disorders.

Causes/Risk Factors: Trauma (blunt or penetrating injuries), blood disorders (such as idiopathic thrombocytopenic purpura), splenic tumors (benign or malignant), or infectious diseases affecting the spleen.

Medical Management: Stabilizing the patient (if traumatic injury), managing underlying conditions, and addressing complications like infection or bleeding before surgery. Vaccinations to prevent post-splenectomy infections are often administered.

Surgical Management: Splenectomy is performed via open surgery or laparoscopic techniques. The surgeon removes the spleen, taking care to control bleeding and prevent damage to surrounding organs.

Prognosis: Patients often experience improved symptoms post-surgery. However, the absence of the spleen increases the risk of certain infections, requiring lifelong preventive measures.

Interesting Fact: After splenectomy, other organs like the liver and bone marrow take over some of the spleen's functions, but the patient needs to be vigilant about infections, especially in the first few years post-surgery.

Splenic Disorders

Definition: Conditions affecting the spleen, including splenomegaly (enlarged spleen), splenic rupture, and splenic abscess.

Pathophysiology: Various causes, including infections, trauma, and underlying systemic diseases.

Signs and Symptoms: Left upper quadrant pain, splenomegaly, anemia, fever.

Causes/Risk Factors: Infections (such as mononucleosis), trauma, liver cirrhosis, and hematologic disorders.

Medical Management: Treatment of underlying cause, pain management, antibiotics for infections.

Surgical Management: Splenectomy (surgical removal of the spleen) in certain cases, such as trauma or specific disorders.

Prognosis: Depends on the specific disorder and its underlying cause.

Interesting Fact: The spleen plays a vital role in the immune system, filtering blood and removing damaged blood cells.

Splenic Rupture

Definition: Tear or rupture of the spleen, often due to trauma, leading to internal bleeding.

Pathophysiology: Blunt or penetrating trauma causes the spleen to rupture, releasing blood into the abdomen.

Signs and Symptoms: Left upper abdominal pain, tenderness, signs of shock.

Causes/Risk Factors: Trauma, such as from car accidents or falls.

Medical Management: Blood transfusion, observation for stable cases.

Surgical Management: Splenectomy (removal of the spleen) for severe or unstable cases.

Prognosis: Depends on the extent of injury and timely intervention; can be life-threatening if untreated.

Interesting Fact: The spleen is vulnerable to injury due to its location and soft consistency.

Splenopexy

Definition: Splenopexy is a surgical procedure that involves fixing a displaced or mobile spleen (splenic ptosis) to its normal anatomical position.

Pathophysiology: In splenic ptosis, the spleen descends from its usual location due to weak or elongated ligaments, predisposing it to torsion, infarction, or trauma.

Signs and Symptoms: Episodic abdominal pain, especially after meals, left upper abdominal tenderness, and a palpable mass in the abdomen.

Causes/Risk Factors: Congenital factors or weakening of the ligaments that hold the spleen in place can lead to splenic ptosis.

Medical Management: Symptomatic relief, pain management, and monitoring for complications. Splenopexy is considered if symptoms are severe or if complications occur.

Surgical Management: During splenopexy, the spleen is repositioned and fixed to its normal position using sutures or mesh. This prevents future displacement.

Prognosis: Splenic function is preserved, and symptoms often improve after splenopexy. Regular follow-ups are essential to monitor the spleen's stability.

Interesting Fact: Splenopexy aims to preserve spleen function while addressing the symptoms associated with a displaced spleen, enhancing the patient's quality of life.

Splenorenal Shunt

Definition: A splenorenal shunt is a surgical procedure performed to treat portal hypertension-related complications by diverting blood flow away from the spleen and reducing the risk of variceal bleeding.

Pathophysiology: Portal hypertension, often due to liver cirrhosis, leads to increased pressure in the portal vein. This can cause varices in the spleen, risking rupture and bleeding.

Signs and Symptoms: Portal hypertension-related complications, such as ascites, splenomegaly, esophageal varices, or signs of bleeding, like melena or hematemesis.

Causes/Risk Factors: Liver cirrhosis, portal vein thrombosis, or other conditions causing increased pressure in the portal vein, leading to complications.

Medical Management: Management of underlying liver disease, medications to reduce portal pressure, and procedures like banding or sclerotherapy for variceal bleeding.

Surgical Management: The splenorenal shunt diverts blood flow away from the spleen, reducing pressure in the splenic veins and preventing variceal bleeding. Different types of shunts can be created surgically.

Prognosis: The procedure helps manage complications of portal hypertension, improving the quality of life and reducing the risk of life-threatening bleeding episodes.

Interesting Fact: Splenorenal shunts are one of the surgical techniques used to alleviate complications of portal hypertension, addressing the underlying cause of variceal bleeding.

Splenorrhaphy

Definition: Splenorrhaphy is a surgical procedure performed to repair a damaged or ruptured spleen, preserving its function.

Pathophysiology: Splenorrhaphy is necessary in cases of splenic trauma, where the spleen is injured but can be salvaged without removal.

Signs and Symptoms: Pain in the left upper abdomen, abdominal tenderness, signs of shock, and a palpable mass in the abdomen due to an enlarged or ruptured spleen.

Causes/Risk Factors: Blunt or penetrating abdominal trauma, such as in car accidents or falls, leading to splenic injuries.

Medical Management: Stabilizing the patient, controlling bleeding and infections, and ensuring hemodynamic stability before surgery. Blood transfusions and intravenous fluids may be administered.

Surgical Management: During splenorrhaphy, the surgeon repairs the damaged spleen, suturing lacerations, and controlling bleeding. Sometimes, a mesh or other supportive materials are used for reinforcement.

Prognosis: If successful, splenorrhaphy preserves the spleen's function and reduces the risk of post-splenectomy complications.

Interesting Fact: Splenorrhaphy is a challenging procedure due to the delicate nature of the spleen tissue, requiring precise surgical techniques to ensure the spleen's integrity post-repair.

Splenosis Resection

Definition: Splenosis is a condition where splenic tissue implants itself in various parts of the abdomen or thorax, often after splenic trauma. Surgical resection may be necessary if it causes symptoms or complications.

Pathophysiology: Splenosis occurs due to autotransplantation of splenic tissue fragments after splenic injury or surgery. These fragments attach to nearby organs and grow, forming nodules.

Signs and Symptoms: Pain, discomfort, or mass formation in the abdomen or thorax, especially if the splenotic nodules compress adjacent structures.

Causes/Risk Factors: Previous splenic trauma or surgery, leading to the dispersion and implantation of splenic tissue fragments.

Medical Management: Symptomatic management, pain relief, and regular monitoring. Imaging studies confirm the presence and location of splenotic nodules.

Surgical Management: Surgical resection of symptomatic splenotic nodules is performed, often requiring meticulous dissection to avoid damage to surrounding organs.

Prognosis: Splenosis resection usually leads to symptom relief and improved quality of life for affected individuals.

Interesting Fact: Splenosis can mimic other conditions, making diagnosis challenging. Surgical removal and histological examination confirm the presence of splenic tissue.

Splenunculi Removal

Definition: Splenunculi are accessory or extra splenic tissue fragments that may cause pain, infection, or other complications, requiring surgical removal.

Pathophysiology: Splenunculi are remnants of the spleen that develop during embryonic development. They can become symptomatic due to inflammation, torsion, or infection.

Signs and Symptoms: Pain or tenderness in the left upper abdomen, especially after meals, recurrent infections, and symptoms of anemia.

Causes/Risk Factors: Congenital factors, such as abnormal embryonic development, lead to the presence of splenunculi.

Medical Management: Managing symptoms, controlling pain, and treating infections if present. Imaging studies confirm the presence and location of splenunculi.

Surgical Management: Surgical removal (splenunculectomy) is performed to excise the accessory splenic tissue, relieving symptoms and preventing complications.

Prognosis: Splenunculi removal typically leads to the resolution of symptoms and improved overall health.

Interesting Fact: Splenunculi are rare and often asymptomatic. However, if they cause symptoms, surgical removal is a safe and effective solution.

Strangulated Hernia

Definition: Hernia in which the blood supply to the trapped tissue is cut off, leading to tissue ischemia.

Pathophysiology: Herniated tissue becomes trapped and loses blood supply.

Signs and Symptoms: Severe pain, redness, swelling, fever, vomiting.

Causes/Risk Factors: Untreated hernia, increased intra-abdominal pressure.

Medical Management: None; requires urgent surgery.

Surgical Management: Hernia reduction and repair, tissue assessment for viability.

Prognosis: Variable; can be life-threatening without prompt intervention.

Interesting Fact: Strangulated hernias are surgical emergencies and can lead to bowel necrosis and sepsis if not treated promptly.

Superior Mesenteric Artery Syndrome (SMAS)

Definition: Compression of the duodenum between the superior mesenteric artery and the aorta, leading to partial or complete obstruction.

Pathophysiology: Narrowing of the space between the vessels, causing duodenal compression.

Signs and Symptoms: Severe abdominal pain, vomiting, bloating, weight loss.

Causes/Risk Factors: Rapid weight loss, prolonged bed rest, scoliosis, prior surgery.

Medical Management: Nutritional support, addressing underlying causes, positioning changes.

Surgical Management: Duodenojejunostomy (surgical bypass of the obstruction) in refractory cases.

Prognosis: Variable, depending on the degree of obstruction and response to treatment.

Interesting Fact: SMAS can cause severe malnutrition and requires a multidisciplinary approach for management.

Surgical Emphysema

Definition: Presence of air in the subcutaneous tissues, often due to surgical or traumatic causes.

Pathophysiology: Air enters the tissues, creating subcutaneous pockets of air.

Signs and Symptoms: Swelling, crepitus (crackling sensation) when touched, pain.

Causes/Risk Factors: Surgical procedures involving the respiratory or gastrointestinal tract, trauma.

Medical Management: Observation for small, non-progressing cases.

Surgical Management: Subcutaneous needle decompression for significant or expanding cases.

Prognosis: Excellent with appropriate management; resolves as the body absorbs the trapped air.

Interesting Fact: Surgical emphysema can occur after certain dental procedures, especially extractions involving the maxilla.

Surgical Site Infection (SSI)

Definition: Infection occurring at the site of a surgical incision or in deep tissues.

Pathophysiology: Bacterial contamination of the surgical site during or after the procedure.

Signs and Symptoms: Redness, swelling, warmth, pain, discharge at the surgical site, fever.

Causes/Risk Factors: Poor surgical technique, compromised immune system, improper wound care.

Medical Management: Antibiotics, wound care, drainage of abscesses if present.

Surgical Management: Debridement of infected tissue, wound exploration, and revision surgery in severe cases.

Prognosis: Variable; can range from mild to life-threatening, depending on the extent of infection.

Interesting Fact: Preventive measures, including proper sterilization and antibiotic prophylaxis, significantly reduce the risk of SSIs.

Thoracic Aortic Aneurysm

Definition: A thoracic aortic aneurysm is an abnormal enlargement of the aorta in the chest, which can lead to life-threatening complications if it ruptures.

Pathophysiology: Weakness in the aortic wall due to genetic factors, atherosclerosis, or conditions like Marfan syndrome, leading to dilation.

Signs and Symptoms: Often asymptomatic; chest or back pain, shortness of breath, coughing, and hoarseness if pressing on nearby structures.

Causes/Risk Factors: Genetic predisposition, hypertension, atherosclerosis, connective tissue disorders, and trauma.

Medical Management: Blood pressure control, lifestyle modifications, and regular monitoring to prevent enlargement.

Surgical Management: Elective surgical repair to prevent rupture; open surgery or endovascular stent grafting.

Prognosis: Prognosis is generally good after successful surgical intervention. Rupture is a life-threatening emergency.

Interesting Fact: Thoracic aortic aneurysms are often silent until they enlarge substantially or rupture, emphasizing the importance of regular screening for high-risk individuals.

Thoracic Endovascular Aortic Repair (TEVAR)

Definition: TEVAR is a minimally invasive procedure to repair aortic diseases, such as aneurysms or dissections, using stent grafts.

Pathophysiology: Aortic aneurysms or dissections weaken the arterial wall, risking rupture.

Signs and Symptoms: Often asymptomatic; incidental findings on imaging studies or symptoms related to aneurysm compression.

Causes/Risk Factors: Atherosclerosis, genetic factors, and hypertension.

Medical Management: Blood pressure control, lifestyle modifications, and surveillance for growth.

Surgical Management: TEVAR, where a stent graft is placed via catheter, reinforcing the weakened aortic section.

Prognosis: The prognosis after successful TEVAR is generally good, reducing the risk of rupture.

Interesting Fact: TEVAR offers a less invasive alternative to open surgery for selected aortic pathologies, reducing recovery time and complications.

Thoracic Outlet Syndrome (TOS)

Definition: TOS is a group of disorders involving compression of blood vessels or nerves in the space between the collarbone and the first rib.

Pathophysiology: Compression of nerves or blood vessels by muscles or an extra rib causes symptoms in the arm and hand.

Signs and Symptoms: Arm pain, numbness, tingling, and weakness, exacerbated by arm movement.

Causes/Risk Factors: Poor posture, trauma, or anatomical abnormalities (extra rib).

Medical Management: Physical therapy, pain management, and lifestyle modifications.

Surgical Management: Surgical decompression of the affected area.

Prognosis: Prognosis varies based on the underlying cause and response to treatment.

Interesting Fact: TOS is more common in women and often affects young adults, especially those involved in repetitive overhead activities.

Thromboangiitis Obliterans (Buerger's Disease)

Definition: Thromboangiitis obliterans is a rare inflammatory condition causing blood vessel blockages in the extremities.

Pathophysiology: Inflammatory changes in blood vessels lead to thrombus formation and arterial occlusion.

Signs and Symptoms: Pain, ulcers, and gangrene in the hands and feet, especially in smokers.

Causes/Risk Factors: Smoking is a major risk factor. Genetic and autoimmune factors may also contribute.

Medical Management: Smoking cessation, medications to improve blood flow, and wound care.

Surgical Management: Sympathectomy and, in severe cases, amputation of affected limbs.

Prognosis: Prognosis is poor without lifestyle changes. Smoking cessation is crucial to prevent disease progression.

Interesting Fact: Thromboangiitis obliterans primarily affects young to middle-aged individuals, especially those with a history of heavy smoking.

Thrombosed Hemorrhoids

Definition: Swollen and inflamed veins in the rectum or anus.

Pathophysiology: Increased pressure in the veins, causing them to swell and become painful.

Signs and Symptoms: Pain, swelling, and bleeding during bowel movements.

Causes/Risk Factors: Straining during bowel movements, constipation, pregnancy.

Medical Management: Topical treatments, dietary modifications, pain management.

Surgical Management: Hemorrhoidectomy (surgical removal of hemorrhoids) for severe cases.

Prognosis: Generally good with appropriate management.

Interesting Fact: Hemorrhoids are a common condition, especially during pregnancy and in older adults.

Thymic Hyperplasia

Definition: Thymic hyperplasia is the enlargement of the thymus gland beyond its normal size.

Pathophysiology: Can be physiological (as seen in children and adolescents) or related to autoimmune diseases, leading to an increase in thymic tissue.

Signs and Symptoms: Often asymptomatic; discovered incidentally during imaging or surgical procedures.

Causes/Risk Factors: Autoimmune diseases (such as myasthenia gravis), infections, and certain genetic factors.

Medical Management: Observation in mild cases, immunosuppressive therapy for autoimmune-related hyperplasia.

Surgical Management: Thymectomy (surgical removal of the thymus gland) in cases associated with autoimmune diseases or when the enlargement causes symptoms.

Prognosis: Prognosis is excellent after surgical removal, especially in cases related to autoimmune disorders.

Interesting Fact: Thymic hyperplasia is often linked to autoimmune conditions like myasthenia gravis, where the immune system mistakenly attacks neuromuscular junctions.

Thymoma

Definition: Thymoma is a rare tumor originating from thymic epithelial cells in the thymus gland.

Pathophysiology: The exact cause is unknown; possibly related to abnormal thymus development or genetic mutations.

Signs and Symptoms: Chest pain, cough, shortness of breath, myasthenia gravis (in some cases), and superior vena cava syndrome if the tumor compresses nearby structures.

Causes/Risk Factors: Unknown, but it is more common in individuals with certain autoimmune diseases.

Medical Management: Surgery is the primary treatment; radiation therapy, chemotherapy, and immunotherapy may be used in advanced cases.

Surgical Management: Surgical resection of the thymus gland (thymectomy), often involving adjacent tissues if the tumor has invaded.

Prognosis: Prognosis varies based on the stage and completeness of resection. Overall, it is relatively good, especially in early-stage tumors.

Interesting Fact: Thymomas are rare, accounting for a small percentage of mediastinal tumors, and can be associated with autoimmune diseases like myasthenia gravis.

Thyroid Cancer

Definition: Malignant tumor in the thyroid gland.

Pathophysiology: Genetic mutations leading to uncontrolled cell growth in the thyroid gland.

Signs and Symptoms: Neck lump, difficulty swallowing, hoarseness, enlarged lymph nodes.

Causes/Risk Factors: Radiation exposure, certain genetic syndromes.

Medical Management: Surgery, radioactive iodine therapy, thyroid hormone replacement.

Surgical Management: Thyroidectomy (removal of the thyroid gland) in most cases.

Prognosis: Generally good, especially for well-differentiated tumors; early detection improves outcomes.

Interesting Fact: Thyroid cancer is often detected incidentally during imaging studies for other conditions and has a high overall survival rate.

Thyroid Disorders

Definition: Conditions affecting the thyroid gland, including hypothyroidism, hyperthyroidism, and thyroid nodules.

Pathophysiology: Imbalance in thyroid hormones (T3 and T4) or abnormal growth of thyroid tissue.

Signs and Symptoms: Fatigue, weight changes, heat/cold intolerance, palpitations, neck swelling.

Causes/Risk Factors: Autoimmune diseases (e.g., Hashimoto's thyroiditis), iodine deficiency, radiation exposure.

Medical Management: Hormone replacement therapy (hypothyroidism), anti-thyroid medications (hyperthyroidism), biopsy for nodules.

Surgical Management: Thyroidectomy (partial or total removal of the thyroid gland) for nodules, cancer, or hyperthyroidism.

Prognosis: Generally good with appropriate management.

Interesting Fact: Thyroid disorders are more common in women, and thyroid nodules are often discovered incidentally during imaging studies.

Thyroid Nodules

Definition: Abnormal growths or lumps in the thyroid gland.

Pathophysiology: Benign or malignant growth due to various factors.

Signs and Symptoms: Often asymptomatic; neck swelling, difficulty swallowing.

Causes/Risk Factors: Iodine deficiency, inflammation, genetic factors.

Medical Management: Thyroid function tests, ultrasound, biopsy for suspicious nodules.

Surgical Management: Thyroidectomy for large nodules, suspicious nodules, or hyperthyroidism.

Prognosis: Variable, depending on the nature of the nodules.

Interesting Fact: Thyroid nodules are common, especially in women and older adults, and most are benign.

Tracheal Stenosis

Definition: Tracheal stenosis is the narrowing of the trachea, often due to prolonged intubation, trauma, or inflammatory conditions.

Pathophysiology: Scar tissue formation in the tracheal wall leads to narrowing of the airway, making breathing difficult.

Signs and Symptoms: Shortness of breath, stridor (high-pitched breathing sound), wheezing, and frequent respiratory infections.

Causes/Risk Factors: Prolonged intubation, trauma to the trachea, Wegener's granulomatosis, or idiopathic causes.

Medical Management: Bronchodilators, corticosteroids, and airway clearance techniques.

Surgical Management: Tracheal resection and anastomosis (surgical removal of the narrowed portion followed by reconnection) or tracheal stenting.

Prognosis: Prognosis depends on the extent and cause of the stenosis. Timely intervention can significantly improve symptoms.

Interesting Fact: Tracheal stenosis can result in life-threatening airway obstruction, necessitating prompt diagnosis and management.

Tracheoesophageal Fistula

Definition: Tracheoesophageal fistula is an abnormal connection between the trachea and esophagus, present from birth.

Pathophysiology: Failure of proper separation between the trachea and esophagus during fetal development, leading to communication between the two structures.

Signs and Symptoms: Difficulty swallowing, coughing or choking during feeding, aspiration, and respiratory distress.

Causes/Risk Factors: Congenital anomaly; often occurs with esophageal atresia (improper development of the esophagus).

Medical Management: Temporary feeding through a gastrostomy tube, and surgical correction in early infancy.

Surgical Management: Surgical repair to close the fistula and reconstruct the esophagus.

Prognosis: Prognosis is excellent after surgical correction. Early intervention ensures proper nutrition and prevents respiratory complications.

Interesting Fact: Tracheoesophageal fistula often require a multidisciplinary team involving neonatologists, pediatric surgeons, and pediatric gastroenterologists for optimal management.

Tuberculosis (Pulmonary Tuberculosis)

Definition: Tuberculosis (TB) is a bacterial infection caused by Mycobacterium tuberculosis, primarily affecting the lungs.

Pathophysiology: Inhalation of airborne TB bacteria leads to infection in the lungs, forming granulomas (tubercles) and potentially spreading to other organs.

Signs and Symptoms: Persistent cough, weight loss, night sweats, fever, hemoptysis (coughing up blood), and fatigue.

Causes/Risk Factors: Close contact with an active TB patient, weakened immune system (HIV/AIDS), malnutrition, and crowded living conditions.

Medical Management: Antituberculosis medications (multiple antibiotics for an extended period), directly observed therapy (DOT), and contact tracing for potential exposures.

Surgical Management: Surgery is rarely necessary but may be considered in cases of drug-resistant TB, large cavities, or complications like hemoptysis.

Prognosis: Prognosis is generally good with appropriate and consistent medical treatment. Early diagnosis and treatment prevent complications and transmission.

Interesting Fact: TB is one of the world's deadliest infectious diseases, but it is curable with proper medical management, including antibiotic therapy.

Varicose Veins

Definition: Swollen, twisted veins, usually in the legs.

Pathophysiology: Weak or damaged valves in the veins cause blood to pool, leading to swelling and discomfort.

Signs and Symptoms: Visible, bulging veins, leg pain, heaviness, itching, cramping.

Causes/Risk Factors: Age, family history, obesity, pregnancy, prolonged standing/sitting.

Medical Management: Compression stockings, leg elevation, exercise. Severe cases may require surgery.

Surgical Management: Vein stripping or endovenous thermal ablation to close off the affected veins.

Prognosis: Generally good with appropriate management.

Interesting Fact: Varicose veins are a common condition, affecting about 10-15% of men and 20-25% of women.

Vascular Trauma

Definition: Vascular trauma involves injuries to blood vessels, often due to accidents or penetrating wounds.

Pathophysiology: Direct injury or laceration causes bleeding, potentially leading to hemorrhage and ischemia.

Signs and Symptoms: External bleeding, swelling, pain, and signs of shock in severe cases.

Causes/Risk Factors: Traumatic events such as accidents, falls, or gunshot wounds.

Medical Management: Immediate stabilization, imaging studies, and blood transfusions if necessary.

Surgical Management: Vessel repair, ligation, or bypass grafting depending on the extent of the injury.

Prognosis: Prognosis varies widely based on the location and severity of the injury. Timely intervention is crucial.

Interesting Fact: Vascular trauma cases often require a multidisciplinary approach involving vascular surgeons, trauma surgeons, and interventional radiologists.

Ventral Hernia

Definition: Herniation of abdominal contents through a weakness or defect in the abdominal wall.

Pathophysiology: Weakened abdominal wall muscles or fascia allow organs or tissues to protrude.

Signs and Symptoms: Visible bulge, discomfort, pain, especially during lifting or straining.

Causes/Risk Factors: Previous abdominal surgery, obesity, pregnancy, heavy lifting.

Medical Management: Supportive garments, lifestyle modifications.

Surgical Management: Hernia repair with mesh, sometimes laparoscopic surgery.

Prognosis: Good with surgical repair; can recur if underlying risk factors are not addressed.

Interesting Fact: Ventral hernias can vary in size and severity, requiring individualized approaches to management.

Volvulus

Definition: Twisting of a portion of the intestine, leading to obstruction and possible ischemia.

Pathophysiology: Intestinal twisting causing obstruction, often related to an anatomic abnormality.

Signs and Symptoms: Abdominal pain, distension, vomiting, constipation.

Causes/Risk Factors: Congenital malformations, adhesions, previous abdominal surgeries.

Medical Management: IV fluids, decompression, sometimes endoscopic detorsion.

Surgical Management: Surgical detorsion, and resection in case of necrosis.

Prognosis: Good with prompt intervention; can be life-threatening if untreated.

Interesting Fact: Volvulus is a medical emergency requiring immediate surgical attention to prevent intestinal necrosis.

Wilms Tumor (Nephroblastoma)

Definition: Malignant kidney tumor primarily affecting children.

Pathophysiology: Uncontrolled cell growth in the kidney tissue, often arising from embryonic cells.

Signs and Symptoms: Abdominal mass, abdominal pain, hematuria, hypertension.

Causes/Risk Factors: Usually sporadic; certain genetic syndromes predispose to Wilms tumor.

Medical Management: Chemotherapy, radiation therapy.

Surgical Management: Nephrectomy, sometimes followed by chemotherapy.

Prognosis: Generally good with early detection and multimodal treatment.

Interesting Fact: Wilms tumor is the most common kidney cancer in children and has a high survival rate with appropriate treatment.

Zenker's Diverticulum

Definition: Outpouching in the mucosa of the esophagus, often occurring above the upper esophageal sphincter.

Pathophysiology: Weakness in the esophageal wall, leading to pouch formation.

Signs and Symptoms: Dysphagia, regurgitation, halitosis, chronic cough, aspiration pneumonia.

Causes/Risk Factors: Age-related weakening of esophageal muscles, and increased pressure during swallowing.

Medical Management: Dietary modifications, speech therapy, endoscopic dilation.

Surgical Management: Diverticulectomy, myotomy, or diverticulopexy.

Prognosis: Excellent with surgical intervention; resolves swallowing difficulties and prevents complications.

Interesting Fact: Zenker's diverticulum can cause significant swallowing difficulties and can lead to malnutrition and aspiration pneumonia if untreated.